AF739903

Experiencing the Body

Experiencing the Body: A Psychoanalytic Dialogue on Psychosomatics offers a range of perspectives on somatic illness, highlighting key points of convergence and difference between a range of psychoanalytic perspectives, to find a new understanding of this important issue.

Each chapter presents contributions from two experienced clinicians who present different points of view, before concluding with commentary from a third. The book features discussion on key theoretical issues, including drive and affects, the role of the ideal ego, and the function of symbolisation, but also includes case studies of somatic patients, covering issues around depression and trauma, and exploring similarities and differences between somatic and borderline patients. Key treatment issues are also described, such as psychosomatic investigation and the issue of transference and countertransference.

The result of a working party on psychosomatics of the European Psychoanalytical Federation, this unique book not only asks whether somatic illness arises from an impoverishment of the psyche or is primarily a form of communication through or by the body, but goes beyond this classical opposition. It will appeal to any psychoanalyst or psychotherapist interested in this contentious and fascinating area.

Jacques Press, coordinator of this collective work, is a teaching and supervising analyst at the Swiss Psychoanalytical Society and Chair of the Working Party on Psychosomatics of the European Psychoanalytical Federation. He was trained by Pierre Marty and Michel Fain and was awarded the Pierre Marty Psychosomatic Award in 1997. He is the author of two books and numerous articles.

Experiencing the Body

A Psychoanalytic Dialogue on Psychosomatics

Jacques Press
Fotis Bobos
Jörg Frommer
Marina Perris-Myttas
Eva Schmid-Gloor
Bérengère de Senarclens
Christian Seulin
Luigi Solano
Nick Temple

Associate Editor Catherine Humble

Routledge
Taylor & Francis Group
LONDON AND NEW YORK

First published 2019
by Routledge
2 Park Square, Milton Park, Abingdon, Oxon OX14 4RN

and by Routledge
52 Vanderbilt Avenue, New York, NY 10017

Routledge is an imprint of the Taylor & Francis Group, an informa business

© 2019 editorial matter, introductory and concluding chapters, Jacques Press; individual chapters, the contributors

The right of Jacques Press to be identified as the author of the editorial material, and of individual chapters, has been asserted in accordance with sections 77 and 78 of the Copyright, Designs and Patents Act 1988.

All rights reserved. No part of this book may be reprinted or reproduced or utilised in any form or by any electronic, mechanical, or other means, now known or hereafter invented, including photocopying and recording, or in any information storage or retrieval system, without permission in writing from the publishers.

Trademark notice: Product or corporate names may be trademarks or registered trademarks, and are used only for identification and explanation without intent to infringe.

British Library Cataloguing-in-Publication Data
A catalogue record for this book is available from the British Library

Library of Congress Cataloging-in-Publication Data
A catalog record has been requested for this book

ISBN: 978-0-367-18155-0 (hbk)
ISBN: 978-0-367-18157-4 (pbk)
ISBN: 978-0-429-05981-0 (ebk)

Typeset in Times New Roman
by Apex CoVantage, LLC

Contents

Notes on contributors vii
Foreword ix
Acknowledgements xi

Introduction 1
JACQUES PRESS

SECTION I
Two cases 9
MARINA PERRIS-MYTTAS, FOTIS BOBOS

SECTION II
Clinical pictures 33

1 **Depression and psychosomatics** 35
JACQUES PRESS, NICK TEMPLE, EVA SCHMID-GLOOR

2 **Trauma and its effects** 47
FOTIS BOBOS, JÖRG FROMMER, BÉRENGÈRE DE SENARCLENS

3 **Somatic and borderline states** 60
BÉRENGÈRE DE SENARCLENS, CHRISTIAN SEULIN,
MARINA PERRIS-MYTTAS

SECTION III
Treatment 71

4 **Psychosomatic investigation and treatment** 73
EVA SCHMID-GLOOR, JACQUES PRESS, CHRISTIAN SEULIN

5 **Transference and countertransference** 83
MARINA PERRIS-MYTTAS, EVA SCHMID-GLOOR, LUIGI SOLANO

SECTION IV
Theoretical issues 97

6 **Drives and affects** 99
MARINA PERRIS-MYTTAS, CHRISTIAN SEULIN, JÖRG FROMMER

7 **Ideal ego, ego ideal and superego** 112
BÉRENGÈRE DE SENARCLENS, NICK TEMPLE, FOTIS BOBOS

8 **Symbolisation** 123
LUIGI SOLANO, FOTIS BOBOS, NICK TEMPLE

9 **Defence mechanisms and levels of integration** 139
LUIGI SOLANO, JÖRG FROMMER, JACQUES PRESS

Conclusion 151
JACQUES PRESS

Index 155

Notes on contributors

Fotis Bobos is a training and supervising analyst and Chair of the Scientific Committee at the Hellenic Psychoanalytical Society. He is a training analyst at the Hellenic Psychosomatic Society and member at the Institut de Psychosomatique Pierre Marty and the Association Internationale de Psychosomatique P. Marty (AIPPM). He has written various articles for Hellenic psychoanalytical journals and books. For many years he has given lectures and supervisions in mental health institutions.

Jörg Frommer is psychosomatist, psychiatrist, and training and supervising analyst at the Deutsche Psychoanalytische Gesellschaft and at the International Psychoanalytical Association (IPA). He received his training at Heidelberg, Homburg, and Düsseldorf. In 1996 he founded the Department of Psychosomatic Medicine and Psychotherapy at the University Hospital in Magdeburg.

Marina Perris-Myttas is a training and supervising analyst of the British Psychoanalytical Society in private practice since 1995. She is a member of the Institut de Psychosomatique Pierre Marty. She has worked extensively in the National Health Service as a Consultant Clinical Psychologist in Psychotherapy (Eating Disorders Services), and she led a service for personality disorders. She has published and presented papers in the UK and internationally.

Jacques Press is a teaching and supervising analyst at the Swiss Psychoanalytical Society and Chair of the Working Party on Psychosomatics of the European Psychoanalytical Federation. He was trained by Pierre Marty and Michel Fain and was awarded the Pierre Marty Psychosomatic Award in 1997. He is the author of two books and numerous articles.

Eva Schmid-Gloor works in private practice in Zürich as a teaching and supervising analyst of the Swiss Psychoanalytical Society. She is Vice President of the European Psychoanalytical Federation from 2012 to 2020. She has published many articles and co-authored a book with Bérengère de Senarclens.

Bérengère de Senarclens works in private practice in Geneva as a training analyst of the Swiss Psychoanalytical Society. She was consultant for the Psychiatric

Institutions of the University of Geneva. She has published various articles in European publications and has co-authored a book with Eva Schmid-Gloor. She is presently Chair of the Liaison Committee of the IPA for Psike (Istanbul).

Christian Seulin, MD, is a training and supervising psychoanalyst of the Paris Psychoanalytical Society (SPP), and member of the IPA. He is former Secretary of the Executive Council of the Training Commission of the SPP and former President of the Lyon group of the SPP. Christian has published more than 50 articles and book chapters and one book. As an editor, he was a member of the Publications Committee of the IPA between 2009 and 2017. He lives and practices in Lyon.

Luigi Solano is a member and training analyst of the Italian Psychoanalytic Society. He is former Professor of Psychosomatics at the Department of Clinical and Dynamic Psychology of the Sapienza University of Rome, where he was Director of a Postgraduate School in Health Psychology. He has published several papers in Italian and International publications, and he is the author and editor of a number of volumes on psychosomatics, health psychology, and clinical psychology.

Nick Temple is a training and supervising analyst of the British Psychoanalytical Society and former President of the Society. He is a Consultant Psychiatrist and former Chairman of the Faculty of Psychotherapy of the Royal College of Psychiatrists. Nick was Chairman of the Tavistock Clinic and Chief Executive of the Tavistock and Portman NHS Trust. He has published papers and chapters on psychosomatic disorders, depression, and totalitarian states of mind.

Associate Editor

Catherine Humble is Associate Lecturer in Literature at Kingston University and University College London. She is former Executive Editor of the *International Journal of Psychoanalysis* and editor of a number of articles on psychoanalysis. Catherine has published several articles and book chapters and is currently completing a monograph.

Foreword

This book is the result of the on-going work, an 'emanation', of the Working Party on Psychosomatics of the European Psychoanalytical Federation that began its journey in 2013. The authors, who are the members of the group, represent six different countries and different schools of thought. They have developed an original working method and consequently an original working process that is faithfully reflected in the structure of the book: each chapter is written by three experts in psychosomatics, one of them is 'a silent observer' who highlights and questions the implicit statements in the writing of his/her colleagues.

The authors describe their work as 'a collective adventure' that presupposes a willingness to exchange and to reflect on the divergences and a capacity to 'suspend' their theoretical frameworks to allow for the connection of diverging viewpoints. In a certain sense we can see here something that parallels with the philosophy of language theorised by Donald Davidson as the 'charity principle': a necessary premise that enables proper communication. In this case the 'charity principle' enables general theories to interact with special theories, and a new epistemological position may be formed, and this is not to be confused with relativism – as Jacques Press states in the Conclusion to this book.

As I continued reading this book and consequently shared in its *adventure*, I was reminded of an anecdote that Karl-Otto Apel mentions at the beginning of his *Die Logosauszeichnung der Menschlichen Sprache.* He recalls that his reflections on the linguistic activity of individuals were triggered by a comment from Karl Popper. Following a lecture by Karl-Otto Apel in which Apel attempted to outline his programme of a pragmatic-transcendental theory of communication, Popper said that it was not necessary to pay so much attention to communication inasmuch as this is what we have in common with animals; rather, what is important in human language are the propositions.

Apel writes that Popper's comment refers to the classical paradigm running through the philosophy of language like a scarlet thread from Aristotle to the referential semantics of Frege. The classical or propositional paradigm is the semantic-logical-referential aspect of the *logos*. Through a panoramic vision of the tradition of *logos*, Apel is able to state that the Platonic root of *logos* was dialogic (logos as language and discourse in conversation); if logos is objectified, it takes the meaning of a proposition, of a true or false statement. The next step is taken by Aristotle, who introduced a distinction between *semantikòs* logos and *apofantikòs* logos. The semantic logos of language must therefore be conceived as having a wider meaning than that of the representative function of language, which would be able to reach the truth. From this point of view, the *apofantikòs* logos is dependent on the *semantikòs* logos, where the latter develops its functions of communicative agreement about the world through dialogue.

I think this point by Apel can be fully applied to the philosophy of the project of the Working Party on Psychosomatics, and it corresponds to the criteria of the Platonic *dialeghestai*. Moreover, the project and the book respond to the philosophy that orients the scientific activity of the European Federation of Psychoanalysis: to connect diverging viewpoints, to tolerate the temporary suspension of reciprocal theoretical frameworks, to cultivate the dialogue, to try to increase knowledge. It is for all these reasons and for the quality of the results obtained that I am very pleased to have the opportunity of promoting this book.

Jorge Canestri
President of the European Psychoanalytical Federation

Acknowledgements

The writing of this book would not have been possible without the continuing support of the Executive of the European Psychoanalytical Federation. We would especially like to thank Serge Frisch, former President of the EPF who gave us the encouragement to start our working party, and we are equally grateful to Jorge Canestri, the current President, for his unfailing interest and help.

Introduction

Jacques Press

This book is the outcome of the collective reflection that has been carried out since 2013 within the working party on psychosomatics of the European Psychoanalytical Federation. The initiative came from three Swiss members of our group. As contacts were made, a group made up of nine analysts from six different societies and countries came to be: a group that seemed very heterogeneous at first. While Fotis Bobos, Jörg Frommer, Marina Perris-Myttas, Luigi Solano, and I, pursued a path largely centred on psychosomatics and the treatment of somatising patients, Eva Schmid-Gloor, Bérengère de Senarclens, Christian Seulin and Nick Temple were primarily interested in borderline states and had found themselves faced with the presence or emergence of somatic illnesses in the context of their practice. However, such heterogeneity actually contributed to the wealth and openness of our exchanges. It brought us together on the basis of a common belief that it was time to tackle the various theoretical approaches in the area of psychosomatics. We were intent from the start on rooting our reflections in clinical work. This is what we undertook from our first meetings onwards, via mutual presentations of clinical situations. Exposing ourselves through our daily clinical practice not only contributed to creating friendly ties in the group and fostering dynamics of exchange and interaction that were respectful of our differences, it also contributed to the formation of a group identity. Such a foundation somehow made up the living fabric that enabled us to make progress. We each had to confront unfamiliar ways of thinking and tolerate differences between us. But we also had to confront and make explicit what was often implicit in our own way of thinking and thereby become more aware of it. Moreover, we quickly realised that while we encountered differences and divergences in our understanding of the material and styles of intervention, we were nonetheless able to meet in a common ground for discussion. The divergences proved more deep-rooted when tackling the underlying theories that supported our different approaches.

A preliminary question arose from the start: how does one define psychosomatics? An initial and minimalist reply would consist in stating that it is defined by its object: i.e. patients suffering from somatic illnesses. But this inevitably leads one to wonder about either the factors that are likely to contribute to the development of such illnesses, or conversely about the factors likely to foster a better psychosomatic balance, yielding a broader definition: psychosomatics is concerned with the individual's psychosomatic equilibrium and with an investigation of the economic and/or symbolic value of somatic illness. These questions were deliberately set aside by Freud, but they were conversely of great interest to numerous authors from the beginnings of psychoanalysis, whether we mention Sándor Ferenczi, Georg Groddeck, or Franz Alexander in the following generation.

Subsequently, several schools of thought developed an interest in psychosomatics, but accounting for them all would greatly exceed this introduction. I will settle for a few brief and invariably limited comments. In France, the work of the authors of the Paris School of Psychosomatics (Pierre Marty, Michel Fain, Michel de M'Uzan and Christian David) had a substantial impact and led Marty to put forward a general model of psychosomatic functioning for human beings (Marty, 1976, 1980). For the Paris School of Psychosomatics, according to Michel de M'Uzan's famous dictum, the somatic symptom is *stupid*, i.e. it never takes on a symbolic value. Conversely, Joyce McDougall, influenced by both Donald Winnicott and Jacques Lacan, develops the notion of archaic hysteria; for her, the somatic symptom does have a meaning, but it pertains to psychic survival rather than sexuality, as is the case in classic hysteria (McDougall, 1989, 1996). The line of thought of the founders of the Paris School has been pursued by the current generation. While Marilia Aisenstein and Claude Smadja reformulate Marty's theory in the context of Freud's late drive theory (Aisenstein, 2006; Smadja, 2011), on my part, and engaging with Winnicott's work, I venture the hypothesis that somatisation could occur in place of a Winnicottian breakdown (Press, 2016).

In contrast with these theses, a series of studies from the Kleinian School couch their hypothesis of organic symbolism as much more radical: somatic illness tallies with a projection of primitive fantasies into the body. Developments stemming from Bion's reflection have subsequently added complexity to this perspective (Bronstein, 2011; Lombardi, 2008; Magnenat, 2016). In Italy, Wilma Bucci, a cognitive scientist with personal experience of psychoanalysis, has worked on the various forms and levels of symbolisation, which has been highly influential (Bucci, 1997; Solano, 2010). In the US, taking personality disorders as his starting point, C.P. Wilson (Wilson, 1989) insists on the role of a merciless superego, while G. Taylor (Taylor, 2010) focuses on the question of affect and trauma. While the conceptual tenets of the American thinkers are very different from and often at odds with those of the Paris School, the conclusions that they reach are not unrelated to the Paris School (Sloate, 2016, pp. 1–52). Lastly, the German School of Psychosomatics has a long history, starting from the beginning of the nineteenth century; their work is impossible to summarise in a few sentences (Frommer, 2013), but let us at least mention Alexander Mitscherlich, who developed his work during the years following the Second World War. According to Mitscherlich's view, somatic illness results from repression in two phases (*zwei-phasige verdrängung*): from the conscious to the unconscious, and from the unconscious to the soma (Mitscherlich, 1966). During the last thirty years, however, psychosomatic research in Germany has shifted away from psychoanalysis, although there has been a certain renewal of interest in psychoanalytical psychosomatics in recent years, for example in the work of Joachim Küchenhoff (Küchenhoff, 2012).[1]

Each of the aforementioned authors (or schools) have worked independently and developed their own theorisations. This state of affairs has led to the creation of actual theoretical ghettos, which has generated formidable hurdles in the development of creative scientific exchange. Granted, some books have brought together works by authors from a variety of orientations (Aisenstein and Aisemberg, 2010; Sloate, 2016). However, these books basically offer a juxtaposition of various points of view. On the premise of this observation, we set a double goal for ourselves. On the one hand, we wanted to better define the points of convergence hidden behind distinct metapsychological theorisations, and on the other hand, we wanted to highlight the fundamental differences and divergences more clearly. Therefore, the point has neither been to write an encyclopaedia, nor to give a comprehensive view of the various existing theories in the field of psychosomatics, rather it has consisted in opening up a dialogue across the exchanges that developed within our group.

A few central questions arise across the book: what is the specificity of psychosomatic description? What can we say about the way in which the course of psychic events influences the psychosomatic balance? Is the psychosomatic perspective we advocate a monistic or a dualistic one? And at a more directly clinical level, how do we understand the influence of the object and the early contingencies of object relations on the psychosomatic equilibrium of each individual? We chose not to discuss these questions in separate chapters because we felt it could result in contradictory discussions involving term by term oppositions, which was unlikely to be productive.

It is worth noting that another aspect gradually took on increasing importance in our exchanges, as well as in the organisation of our workshops during the annual conferences of the European Psychoanalytical Federation. I am referring to the attention paid to the specific modalities of transference and countertransference in these clinical cases. Initially, indeed, our meetings and workshops involved two stages. The first stage consisted of the examination of a patient's first interviews, which led us to form some preliminary idea about the patient's modalities of functioning and potential areas of psychosomatic fragility, along with the first transferential and countertransferential dynamics. The second stage focused on the discussion of recent sessions, which reflected the progress of the therapeutic relationship and the ways in which the transferential-countertransferential dynamics had developed. But it quickly dawned on us that questions of transference and countertransference required very special attention, which led us to introduce two new elements to the organisation of our workshops. First, we set up a third stage, where we investigated how hidden transferential-countertransferential issues were reflected in the group dynamics.

Second, we allocated the position of 'silent observer' to a workshop. The 'silent observer' would remain silent most of the time and would only speak at key moments when it was relevant to foreground significant aspects of the dynamics at work in the group, and how such group dynamics might reflect important elements of the transference and countertransference.

It is no overstatement to claim that the present volume has been shaped by these various aspects of our working party: the grounding in clinical practice, the wish for clarification and dialogue between different schools of thought, the attention paid to the transference and the countertransference. Such aspects firstly encouraged us to choose a ternary form for this volume, echoing back something of the structure of our workshops and exchanges. Each chapter focuses on an important topic in psychosomatics such as depression, symbolisation, trauma; and in a rather unorthodox way, the chapters are made up of three parts. To begin with, in each chapter, two authors offer their perspective on the topic under discussion. Then a third contributor, the commentator – an avatar of the 'silent observer' in our workshops – discusses the two viewpoints, at times challenging them, and striving to account for their visible and less visible divergences and convergences. Bringing a third eye to bear on things, the commentator opens up a new space, putting the two authors' contributions in perspective and shedding a new light on them. We hope that such an approach might allow the reader to delve deeply into the ongoing clinical and theoretical issues raised in each chapter.

We also decided to open the book with the presentation of two clinical situations which form the starting point of reflections in subsequent chapters. First, Marina Perris-Myttas describes the case of a patient, Jasmine, whose initial wish for analysis seems too obvious to her analyst and brings about an intense work in her countertransference. This patient displays a dramatic somatic manifestation on the first day that her analysis is supposed to begin, foreshadowing increasingly alarming somatic outbreaks. The case of the second patient, Cate, presented by Fotis Bobos, is very different: when this patient consults the analyst, she is already suffering from breast cancer and the side effects of chemotherapy. Yet as becomes clear, this patient calls upon the countertransference of her analyst with no less intensity. Though they suffer from very different somatic pathologies – illnesses of a limited kind on the one hand, and cancer on the other – these two patients raise many questions that we tackle over the course of the chapters of the book, especially the question of whether a link can be established between the psychic functioning of each of them and the type of somatisations they present. As the reader will surmise, the answer is far from unequivocal. Let us be clear that our aim is not to write a book of commentary pertaining to the two presentations. Rather, the cases operate for the authors and readers alike as a backdrop (more or less explicitly, but always actively) for the topics under discussion in each chapter, and as a uniting thread underlying them.

On the basis of this clinical grounding, the issue was to choose topics we especially wanted to discuss. Here, too, we opted for an approach moving from the clinical to the theoretical. Section I of the book opens with the two clinical cases. Section II: 'Clinical pictures', consists of three chapters that explore some important aspects of the clinical spectrum encountered in the psychosomatic practice. Chapter 1, 'Depression and psychosomatics', examines the role of depression in psychosomatics. First, in my contribution to this chapter, I challenge the central importance bestowed on essential depression in the psychosomatic theory of the Paris School. I insist on the importance of the dynamics of flight before a threat of breakdown in Winnicott's sense, as he sees this at work in the case of Cate. Second, reflecting on the clinical presentations as well as his own practice, Nick Temple links depression to a projection into the body of an unprocessed conflict with an internal object. The contrasts between these two positions and their clinical consequences are at the heart of Eva Schmid-Gloor's discussion.

Chapter 2, 'Trauma and its effects', is devoted to the question of trauma and its effects. First, Fotis Bobos stresses the disorganising impact of early traumas on the psychosomatic equilibrium in light of the two clinical presentations. He suggests that the ego might find itself cut off from its drive-related sources, and so the ego's sole resource would consist in getting its energetic supply from perception, which accounts for the tendency to cling on to the perceptual sphere as is often observed in somatising patients. For his part, Jörg Frommer discerns 'too much excitation' in somatising patients, combined with 'not enough' symbolisation. He insists on the traumatic role of the somatic illness itself, which he sees at work in the case of Cate, and on the analyst's need to bear this aspect in mind. In her discussion, Bérengère de Senarclens foregrounds the difference between the two authors' understandings of the interconnection between external and internal traumatic factors. She asks whether somatisation might convey a call for help for psychic reworking.

Chapter 3, 'Somatic and borderline states', contrasts borderline and somatising states. While highlighting their likeness, Bérengère de Senarclens tends to distinguish them, and locates the borderline state on the side of the avatars of anality, while somatising states pertain more closely to melancholia. Drawing on the work of Jean Bergeret, André Green and Otto Kernberg, Christian Seulin goes on to envisage somatic illnesses as stemming from moments of weakening of the soma against a backdrop of borderline functioning. In her commentary, Marina Perris-Myttas furthers the discussion by opposing acting-out in external reality with acting-in in the soma. She raises the question of the potentially symbolic value of these different forms of acting. And she asks whether the differences reflect differences in the early relationship to the primary object.

Section III focuses on treatment. In Chapter 4, 'Psychosomatic investigation and treatment', Eva Schmid-Gloor uses her experience with borderline patients and the types of somatisation encountered in them as her starting point. She underlines the key role of the countertransference and carries out a detailed examination of her place in the treatment of Jasmine. I myself revisit the notion of psychosomatic investigation, which plays a central role in the theory of the Paris School, before considering the modalities of the treatment. Both of us distance ourselves from the fundamentally diagnostic aim of psychosomatic investigation in the Paris School. In his discussion, Christian Seulin, following René Roussillon, suggests that such investigations be looked at as borderline psychoanalytic situations, and he argues that choosing a clinical setting is a highly individual decision made on a case-by-case basis.

Chapter 5, 'Transference and countertransference', delves deeper into this line of thought. Marina Perris further stresses the key role of the countertransference when working with psychosomatic patients. As for the transference, Marina believes it stops operating precisely at the time of the emergence of somatisation, which she reads as a process of de-psychicisation of the drive, i.e. the drive loses its psychic quality and returns to its somatic origin. Referring in part to a clinical example taken from her own practice, Eva Schmid-Gloor argues that an important countertransferential tool for working with somatising patients is 'thinking with the body', which refers back to the point that somatic symptoms might often consist in a pre- or infra-verbal form of communication. In his commentary, Luigi Solano underlines the point that both authors explore transference and countertransference from opposite yet non-contradictory perspectives: Marina foregrounds the 'speechless mind', while Eva focuses on sensory forms of communication through a 'communicating body'.

Section IV: 'Theoretical issues', revisits some of the theoretical issues that are fundamental to psychosomatics. In Chapter 6, 'Drives and affects', Christian Seulin questions the value of the notion of the death drive in the psychosomatic field. Marina Perris, on the other hand, compares Bion's notion of beta-elements with the concept of drive, arguing that because the drive implies a rooting in the soma it has a heuristic value in understanding somatisation processes which Bion's theory lacks. In his discussion, Jörg Frommer argues that the drive concept retains a metaphorical value but is obsolete as a biological explanatory notion.

Chapter 7, 'Ideal ego, ego ideal and superego', opposes two viewpoints – those of Bérengère de Senarclens and Nick Temple respectively – of the notions of ideal and superego, and their place in psychosomatics. Could somatic illness result from a disintegration of the ego subjected to exorbitant ideal demands? Or does it stem from an unprocessed conflict with an archaic superego that is manifested in the body? Fotis Bobos's subtle discussion detects points of convergence underlying these apparently conflicting theorisations.

In Chapter 8, 'Symbolisation', Luigi Solano draws on Wilma Bucci to present a detailed account of his view of symbolisation processes. He argues that they convey not only a demand for work on the part of the psyche, but also a primary form of bodily language, initially devoid of symbolic value and awaiting transformation through the presence of the object. For his part, Fotis Bobos engages with Roussillon's distinction between primary symbolisation and secondary symbolisation as his starting point. He suggests that the role of the analyst is to work along the symbolisation spectrum from the bodily aspects to the symbolic system of language. Both authors base their thoughts on a detailed examination of the clinical work carried out with Cate and Jasmine. In his commentary, Nick Temple underlines the links between the two authors' ideas and he ventures the hypothesis that defences against primitive anxieties might interfere with the symbolisation processes.

Chapter 9, 'Defence mechanisms and levels of integration', shows the specificity of the psychosomatic approach: it forces us to envision the psychosomatic construction not only in terms of defence mechanisms, but as levels of functioning of increasing complexity. Luigi Solano argues that the more that integration is problematic, the more radical the defence mechanisms will be. For his part, Jörg Frommer resorts to semiotics to reflect on these various levels of psychosomatic functioning. In my discussion, I question the absence of the economic viewpoint – a fundamental one, in my view – in my colleagues' elaborations. Finally, in the Conclusion, I draw lessons from the collective adventure of writing this book.

Not offering a ready-made theory of psychosomatics but comparing and contrasting various modes of thinking and theoretical frames; amending our way of working without foregoing our own frame of references; being led, as a result, to new points of question and at times to new paths. Such was our project, such was our journey as well. This is equally what we wish for our readers: that the dialogues opened up by this book should broaden their horizons and foster new pathways; that our readers may be led to create their own personal theory; that, finally, they should be in a position to better grasp the complexity of psychosomatic reflections and the enrichments they provide, not only for a limited group of specialists but for anyone interested in psychoanalysis.

Addendum: some remarks on terminology

As is hardly surprising in a book written by nine people coming from six psychoanalytic societies, six countries and speaking five different languages, we had to face issues of translation on two levels: the translation from one language to another and from one school to another. For example, the terms 'psychicisation' (*psychisation*) or 'qualification/disqualification' of affects (*qualification/déqualification*) are commonly used in Francophone psychoanalytic literature, whereas they are rare in English-speaking scholarship. Obviously, the issue is not strictly a linguistic one, insofar as the use of these terms underlies the use of a theoretical framework of the drive, with excitation going from the somatic to the psychic. Other terms are used in a very different sense from one language to another. The term 'mentalisation' is thus used by Pierre Marty to account for the quality of mental functioning, especially the quality of preconscious functioning, whereas in the aftermath of Peter Fonagy's work it has taken on a very distinct connotation in the Anglophone psychoanalytic world. To avoid any confusion, we strove to avoid the term 'mentalisation' as much as possible. Lastly, the French phrase *pensée (ou vie) opératoire* is a real challenge to any translator. We ultimately chose to translate it as 'operative life'.

Note

1 I thank Jörg Frommer for his information about psychosomatics in Germany.

References

Aisenstein, M. (2006) 'The indissociable unity of psyche and soma: a view from the Paris Psychosomatic School', *Int. J. Psychoanal.*, 87, pp. 667–80.
Aisenstein, M. and Aisemberg, E.R. (2010) *Psychosomatics Today: A Psychoanalytical Perspective*. London: Karnac.
Bronstein, C. (2011) 'On psychosomatics: the search for meaning', *Int. J. Psychoanal.*, 92, pp. 173–95.
Bucci, W. (1997) *Psychoanalysis and Cognitive Science: A Multiple Code Theory*. New York: Guilford Press.
Frommer, J. (2013) 'Contemporary perspectives on psychosomatics in Germany: A comment on Karin Gubb's paper "Psychosomatics today: a review of contemporary theory and practice"', *The Psychoanalytic Review*, 100, pp. 157–68.
Küchenhoff, J. (2012) *Körper und Sprache: Theoretische und klinische Beiträge zu einem intersubjektiven Verständnis des Körpererlebens* [Body and language: The theoretical and clinical contributions to an intersubjective understanding of bodily experience]. Giessen: Psychosozial.
Lombardi, R. (2008) 'The body in the analytic session: focusing on the body–mind link', *Int. J. Psychoanal.*, 89, pp. 89–120.
McDougall, J. (1989) *Theatres of the Body: Psychoanalytic Approach to Psychosomatic Illness*. London: Free Association Books.
McDougall, J. (1996) *The Many Faces of Eros: A Psychoanalytic Exploration of Human Sexuality*. New York: Norton & Co.
Magnenat, L. (2016) 'Psychosomatic breast and alexithymic breast: a Bionian psychosomatic perspective', *Int. J. Psychoanal.*, 97, pp. 41–63.
Marty, P. (1976) *Les mouvements individuels de vie et de mort*. Paris: Payot.
Marty, P. (1980) *L'ordre psychosomatique*. Paris: Payot.
Mitscherlich, A. (1966) *Die krankheit als konflikt*. Frankfurt: Suhrkampf Verlag.
Press, J. (2016) 'Metapsychological and clinical issues in psychosomatics research', *Int. J. Psychoanal.*, 97, pp. 89–113.
Sloate, P.L. (ed.) (2016) *From Soma to Symbol: Psychosomatic Conditions and Transformative Experience*. London, Karnac.
Smadja, C. (2011) 'Psychoanalytic psychosomatics', *Int. J. Psychoanal.*, 92, pp. 221–30.
Solano, L. (2010) 'Some thoughts between body and mind in the light of Wilma Bucci's multiple code theory', *Int. J. Psychoanal.*, 91, pp. 1445–64.
Taylor, G.J. (2010) 'Symbolism, symbolization, and trauma in psychosomatic theory', in M. Aisenstein, and E.R. Aisemberg (eds), *Psychosomatics Today: A Psychoanalytical Perspective*. London: Karnac.
Wilson, C.P. (1989) 'Family psychopathology', in C.P. Wilson and I.L. Mintz (eds), *Psychosomatic Symptoms: Psychodynamic Treatment of the Underlying Personality Disorder*. Northvale, NJ: Jason Aronson.

Section I

Two cases

Clinical case: Jasmine

Marina Perris-Myttas

Part I: First consultation

Jasmine arrived for her first consultation a few minutes late. She was visibly rushed and in a hurry. I felt her sense of urgency, which soon disappeared without a trace. Jasmine settled comfortably into the consultation and talked about herself with ease. The first thing she told me was related to her 'wish' to have an analysis. 'I often have the feeling that I should be more pleased with my life, instead I often have a sense of futility, a sense of "what's next"'. I noticed that hers was a 'wish' to be in analysis not a 'necessity' of any description.

Jasmine was an intelligent, attractive and accomplished professional woman, a successful lawyer, in her mid-forties. She was in a 'difficult but fulfilling marriage' and happy as a mother of her daughters aged six and four. She was herself the youngest of four children, two older sisters and a brother closer to her age – five years older than her. I heard details of her early life in what was presented as 'a loving, supportive family'. Her narrative progressed in a coherent way. She was emotionally present and reflective. She talked a lot about her father and about a special closeness with him which 'she had enjoyed all her life'. There was no sense of oedipal pain resulting from the dissolution of the oedipal complex, or of triumph. She was 'the apple' of her father's eye, almost naturally, it seemed.

While she was talking about herself and her father, the following thought formed in my mind: I thought that the 'affinity' to her father was linked to a feeling, which she and him shared, that there was something the matter with 'mother's love'. I also noticed that she was speaking as if she was an only child. When I shared my observation with her, she momentarily looked puzzled and even troubled; but then very quickly, as if recuperated, she gave me an account of her siblings. All three were quite older than herself. She spoke of their achievements and accomplishments. Nothing much transpired except her understanding that 'they did not like me very much because I was my father's favourite'. Then, she added, that was truer of her sisters than of her brother.

She talked about how she and her brother became closer from adolescence onwards: they had the same political ideas and were going out with each other's social groups. He was, however, at times critical and aggressive. They had fights. She became alive when, in response to my observation that they 'shared things', she talked about how they often shared 'private jokes' when friends were present and how she never knew whether that was pleasurable or embarrassing for herself and even more so for him.

Jasmine regarded herself as sociable; she did well and enjoyed her education. She told me that she had a series of boyfriends over the years, but the quality of her love life was quite obscured. She got married in her late twenties with a man she was and remained in love with, she said.

I had the sense that Jasmine spoke freely and eloquently in long stretches; she gave me an articulate and rather touching account of her life. For the most part during this first consultation, while I did have moments where I noticed incongruities and became aware of pain in her, or even felt an evocation of something quite troubling and inaccessible, I was in the main perplexed with how often the thought came to my mind, 'what does this articulate, thoughtful woman need an analysis for?'

I was still left with this question at the end of the first meeting; and it was only during the second consultation that I was able to make sense of my reaction. Towards the end of the consultation, and as we were fixing our next meeting, I noticed again the urgency I felt that was present in the beginning. She quickly took out her diary and readily agreed with the day I suggested. Then the tempo of her reaction slowed down as if she was resuming her composure, she thanked me and left; she was relieved, I felt.

After the session, I remembered how she had started by telling me about her 'wish' to be in analysis and I had the thought that maybe she was looking to the analytic relationship as such to give her something that she 'wishes for'.

Second consultation

For the second meeting, she came on time. She started with silence and after few minutes she said: 'So can we please discuss what times you might have available. I have been thinking since we last met, and I have decided that I do wish to start my analysis'. She spoke in a matter-of-fact way. I thought she was concerned and rather sad, but not worried about her situation. I thought to myself that she had decided to have an analysis for rather 'preventive' reasons. I said something to that effect. She remained silent then she nodded slightly and made eye-contact for a brief moment and her eyes welled up. I felt that my observation had almost hurt her.

She remained silent and then proceeded to talk about her life for some time. It was mostly about her professional life. She was thoughtful but I was increasingly feeling as if my presence was irrelevant to her. Halfway into this second interview my question, 'what does she need the analysis for', again came into my mind. So I told her at some point that she seemed quite clear about making sense of her past and present experiences, and that this clarity included, in an almost paradoxical way, her decision announced at the very beginning of the consultation that she had decided to start psychoanalysis with me. She responded, 'I like you and want to work with you, it is mostly about this feeling of futility that descends on me: everything becomes grey, it makes me almost feel unwell'.

This was poignantly said, but no sooner had the thought and feeling been brought between us, she shifted; the thought was left behind and she continued talking, about her life, her years in law school, a time that was 'fun and good in terms of work'.

This shift was done in a distinctly autonomous manner, I thought; I felt that it was very important for her to impress her independence upon me, even more so after my last intervention, which I felt had brought about a brief moment of her vulnerability in the context of the emotional contact between us. As Jasmine continued to talk in her articulate and independent manner, I came to realise that the recurrence of my question was a sign of my countertransference response to her.

I was becoming more and more aware, as the session proceeded, that my questioning was the manifestation of my identification with an object now internal, who considered her self-sufficient and certainly not in need of anything coming from the other. I was then drawn to conform to her unconscious communication to regard her as able and autonomous thus actualising the nature of her object.

By the end of this consultation a distinct thought became clear to me: I had to stay actively aware of her unconscious call – to perceive her as very well able to stand on her own two feet – if I were to make it possible for her to engage in the analysis she was asking for and which, by that time, I knew she needed. Further, this thought of mine was an early signal of her sense of precariousness and fragility, which we came to experience in later years of analysis.

Towards the end of this second session I let her know that we had little time left. She responded by trying to speak again about her wish for analysis in the matter of fact way that I'd noticed in her first session. I felt, however, that by the end of this session she was closer to communicating her distressed state. She spoke about her desperation when she felt 'unappreciated' in her life, her despair about feeling 'quite undone' when people didn't welcome and like her. As she spoke about this, a feeling of melancholy became present. She also talked, almost as if in parenthesis, about of 'losing it' at times, resorting to outbursts of rage during which she felt an 'almost compulsion to undo my life in fury'. At these times she feared that she stood to lose 'all that mattered' to her. Her communication was marked by a double aspect: she communicated her pain, and yet her thoughts were related to me almost as 'presenting symptoms', rather than as external to herself.

I thought at that point that I knew little about her mother, and I noticed the timing of this thought. It followed from my having been impressed by her sense, which conveyed a great fear I felt, that she could lose 'all that mattered'. Was this very early 'loss' connected to her mother, the recurrence of which she felt threatened by?

Indeed, the depth of her vulnerability emerged some years later and presented itself outside her psychic field through the process of somatisation or acting-in the body, as it has been called (Aisenstein, 2006). On the eve of the day that her analysis was due to start, Jasmine developed an acute abdominal pain. 'The pain was lethal', she told me when she arrived for her first session a week later than the planned starting date.

'Last week', she explained, she was 'rushed' to the emergency room. She was kept overnight for investigations. Medical tests were still going on. These investigations filled her, and the first days of her analysis, with worries and uncertainty, still expressed in a rather subtle way. This picture was short-lived, a 'transient episode' she said, since by the end of the first week she was told that there was 'no reason for concern on medical grounds'. Soon the 'episode' was forgotten. This opening gesture, however, proved to be a pointer to the shape of things to come: a leap of the somatic into her psychic world, which happened a few years into the analysis and which was neither transient nor subtle.

Memories: the maternal lineage

Jasmine had a difficult relationship with her mother. She thought that 'objectively' her mother was giving and devoted to her children, but more so to her sisters and brother than her. Jasmine remembered that as she was growing up, she had 'explained' this to herself by thinking that she had arrived 'late' for her mother, and for that reason she was not welcome. The mother had herself told Jasmine that she was not expecting to have another baby. She had thought her family was already complete when she 'found' herself pregnant with her.

The mother had her first baby girl when she was 19. She was anxious and uneasy in her mothering. For instance, as a young child Jasmine heard the following story. Her mother was in the kitchen holding her few months old baby (the patient's oldest sister) in her arms. The kitchen stove caught fire. The mother felt paralysed and could not move; she would not leave the kitchen. A couple of neighbours came to help and tried to persuade the mother to hand them the baby so that she, herself, would be freer to move. She refused any help and remained immobilised for some time before she slowly managed to move away. She then explained to the neighbours that she did not want to part from her baby because if she were to come to harm it would be better for the baby to share her fate rather than have a life 'without a mother'. This story was the mother's attempt to speak about how her fear that she and her baby were in danger was so unbearable that it paralysed her mind and made her think and behave 'like a mad woman'.

Jasmine had no memory of her mother's physical affection. Her memory of the absence of affection was more present and painful around the times when she had fallen ill as a child. She remembered the times when she had colds or 'tummy aches' during her primary school years. She would stay at home in bed. She remembered feeling very lonely. Her mother would come in her room only to bring food, or would open the door to ask, 'Are you feeling better?', or 'Are you going to school tomorrow?' She felt that her mother could not 'stand her' being ill.

The maternal grandmother was very present during her early childhood. Jasmine described her as giving but also mainly as critical and harsh. She had a memory, which had the quality of a screen memory, from when she was five or six. She remembered her grandmother walking into the dining room where she was dancing and singing in front of the mirror. She remembered that she was singing 'fair little ladies dancing in a rose-garden'. In her mind she was a 'little lady', dancing. She remembered the pleasure she felt. Her grandmother closed the door behind her and left without saying anything. Feeling embarrassed, she stopped her dancing and followed her grandmother into the kitchen where she overheard her talking to her mother, 'what's wrong with this girl? Dancing in front of the mirror like this?' Jasmine walked away. She remembered having been baffled and ashamed: 'I felt my mother was put to shame as well and that was even harder to bear', she told me.

Jasmine vividly remembered her own fantasies and dialogues with herself. As a young child, she had the following repetitive daydream. She would be hit by a car in a street not far from home, and she would die on the spot. Her family, mainly her mother, would hear what had happened. Her mother would drop whatever she was doing and run to the site of the accident: she would be out of control, distraught, crying and screaming. At times, the fantasy would stop there. Her mother was left in a state of emotional pain and disbelief, but at the same time thinking: 'This serves her right'. She would then have a sense of relief.

At other times the fantasy had a second, calmer scene: the actual funeral. This would be a time of overwhelming sadness for all the family. In this second scene she would witness her family's devastation and would be moved to tears. There is one last story I want to mention. This story was told to her by her five-years-older cousin when they were both grown up. In their young age the two girls were great friends. Jasmine retold me this story after the sessions I will be presenting below.

Her cousin remembered herself to be curious and excited, visiting the hospital a few days after baby Jasmine was born. When they arrived, Jasmine's mother was holding her new-born baby in her arms, standing by the window. A street festival was going on and they all watched it together. The cousin thought that her aunt was very happy. An atmosphere of great excitement was conveyed.

When they left, however, her cousin remembered being angry and telling her mother; 'Aunt Catherine is a liar, all this time she was complaining and cross about having to have another baby, and now she is all happy!'

The memory of this story had first arrived early in analysis, and returned after the period of her illness, to be reworked, I thought. It became pivotal in the deepening of our understanding of her representation of her maternal object, her struggle to identify with and to cathect it. Processes which taken together shaped the development of her femininity.

Part II: Analysis

Over the first years we were, at times, tracing other short-lived occurrences of somatisation. At those times, what was communicated in a condensed manner through the very first bodily gesture – the 'lethal pain' on the eve of her first analytic session – was coming into focus and we were able to explore its multiple psychic dimensions. I shall come back to this later.

The clinical material presented here belongs in the sixth year of Jasmine's analysis when somatic processes emerged and took centre stage for quite some time. In order to put the material in context, I will briefly describe what transpired just before the beginning of the somatisation.

By the end of the sixth year Jasmine had grown in all areas of her life and she was almost free of spells of desperation. She was fond of her analysis and a positive transference, albeit coloured by idealisation, was the affective background of the analytic work. The painful feelings of not being invited and included had lost their intensity and she was less frequently 'under their spell'.

In the last couple of years, however, negative transference had become an increasingly present undercurrent in her feelings for me. Idealisation became more present at the same time, in a defensive manner a stance which, given her narcissistic fragility, made her negative feelings rather difficult to access through analytic work.

The period of somatisation

For some time before the period of somatisation there was a slight shift, in that I was increasingly experiencing the presence of a rather persistent irritation and frustration, which we started to be able to focus on. Furthermore, Jasmine's negative feelings had a new quality; she was conveying a sense of mute discontent, and often I was aware of resigned disappointment in her analyst. I was developing a sense of inadequacy and I had the feeling that this was not only and not even primarily the product of identification with my patient's failing internal object (Racker, 1957), but that it also had to do with something happening in the analysis itself, in the transference and mostly in the countertransference, which was not accessible as yet.

At that time Jasmine started developing an increasingly close relationship with Mr K, a friend of hers from her past, and the friendship became intimate in an exciting way but was never a sexual affair. It was in this context that Jasmine started developing somatic symptoms. She became increasingly stressed, exhausted, and pervasively anxious. She first developed severe tinnitus, 'a loud noise' she called it, which when investigated was diagnosed as functional, but very quickly became the focus of hypochondriacal ideation.

Following the investigations for the tinnitus which was not found to have an organic basis and was attributed to 'stress', she developed a difficulty in controlling hypertension and tachycardia, which together with the persistent and intensifying tinnitus, dominated her life and at times paralysed her functioning. She would often have to miss work, as she was too anxious about having to 'concentrate all day': she would just stay home and come to analysis.

During that period all her feelings were replaced by anxiety. Her attempts to make sense of her experiences, including the transference, were virtually non-existent, and my attempts to explore with her this state of mind seemed fruitless. In her sessions she was endlessly preoccupied with possible bodily ailments: she was bringing her body to me constantly in a torturous manner. Apart from these agonising preoccupations, this was a period of extensive silence which became, at the time, all I had to listen to.

I did experience this development as the way in which her 'mute discontent' was manifesting itself in analysis. Its unfolding, I thought, was following the path of a somatic regression. A few months later the somatic regression had crystallised into a new persistent symptom: she started developing recurrent cysts in her breast. With this new problem Jasmine was filled with the need to actually be in my presence: she felt that the physical proximity with me was keeping her safe. 'Death', she used to say, 'could not catch her' when she was at my side. The threat caused by the physically absent object was then palpable.

Our previous analytic work allowed her to revisit the threat that the absent object creates. All the same, the dread of breast cancer and the terror of an imminent death became her constantly agonising preoccupation. Worrying investigations by doctors came out negative and Jasmine's alleviation of anxiety was temporary only until the next cyst and the next terror of cancer.

This was a period of great distress. I was struggling: at times identifying with her pain, at times sensing that I was failing to comprehend and 'free' her from her agony. Staying with her feelings and elaborating my own, with time, took us to a place where the punishing nature of her experiences to herself and to me, as well as their function as a retreat into a narcissistic state of mind where there was no object to injure or offend her, could be explored. This work generated a significant movement away from the hypochondriacal preoccupations that had flooded the analysis. However, the recurrence of the cysts persisted.

During that period, she was also preoccupied with her relationship with Mr K in a way that paralleled the intensities in the transference: how, she was asking herself, did she allow 'it' to happen? To get so close to a man without ensuring that he already wanted her. She was never sure if he had sexual feeling for her. She felt tantalised. Looking back at her life she was then coming to the awareness that she was flirting only when she felt sure that she was already desired and that the relationship would develop into a sexual one. I was feeling her painful longing in the transference.

She was coming to the sessions without fail, often exhausted and most of the times in a state of panic.

First session: Monday

(During the previous week she had investigated the fourth cyst which her doctor had initially thought to be alarming. She had cancelled her Friday session, as she had an appointment for a second opinion related to this cyst.)

Jasmine arrived on time and looked at me, a fleeting eye-contact as she was lying on the couch.

Jasmine: It is just more waiting, she said in a rush.

Then a long pause.

A: And there was a longer wait than usual for your session today.

Jasmine: I had to make Dr L's appointment. On Friday, I did think that I would be more anxious if I did not come to my session, but I panicked in the end I felt I had to see him.

Long pause.

He aspirated the cyst and said that if the aspiration turns out positive, if there are cancerous cells, I will probably need an operation. 'Partial', did he say? Did he mean a mastectomy? I left without asking, in panic. What does it mean partial? I almost left running and I thought of calling you.

Long pause.

A: You were in too much panic to come to your session for us to try and understand it and then you are left with needing me to know what is happening in your body.

Jasmine: I had the image that I was grabbing your arm [she raises her arms above her head to show me] like that, with my two fists, squeezing you.

Long pause.

She talked about the weekend doing things with her daughters, going to the theatre with her husband and friends; I was 'like an automaton'.

She went on saying that 'If he (Dr L) says it is positive, I will have another opinion before I decide what to do'. She kept talking, developing in the process a paralysing fear about her survival.

It was towards the end of the session and I said to Jasmine that she wanted the doctors and the 'doctor' in me to look at her body, examine her breast again and again; and that maybe it was easier to ask them to look than longing for me to do so. There was a pause, and I added, 'And this longing fills you with panic especially on the Friday in which you missed your session'.

She made no response. A long silence followed before it was time to finish.

Tuesday

She arrived ten minutes late and went straight to the couch without looking at me. She quickly said that she was almost 'ill' with anxiety and pain in her breast. She had vertigo and she had not been able to go to work. After some silence, she started talking with long pauses. This lasted throughout the session. She did indeed talk very little, mostly trying to speak to me of how ill she felt. She gave details of moving around her house and her efforts to speak with friends; she was trying to find a breast surgeon who she could 'trust' to have a third opinion if she were to need it. Her communications to me were filled with confusion. At some point she stopped talking and there was a long silence.

I found myself struggling to stay with her anxiety and follow her thoughts. I had in my mind my interpretation of the last session. I knew it had affected her and I wanted to wait to find myself in a place with clearer visibility before I was to attempt to get back to it.

When she spoke again, she referred to 'this sharp pain' in her breast.

A: I was just reminded that you had used this expression 'sharp pain' before; a few months ago, when you worried about your heart. The sharp pain then was always followed by your heart beating fast, like being excited.

She interrupted me in an almost eager manner, 'Yes, and that was making me anxious'. There was a long pause and she continued, 'it is the same kind of anxiety'.

Wednesday

She arrived on time and went to the couch quickly, avoiding the possibility of eye-contact.

Jasmine: I never stopped being anxious yesterday. I shall hear from Dr L tomorrow. I went to bed late, I slept OK, though I had a dream that I remember. I do not know the last time I remembered a dream.

I was waking up in a room, a living room or bedroom. It was a heavy and darkish place. I sensed K's presence nearby. He was lying down on a bed, a sofa, he had his eyes shut. I think he was asleep. I felt alarmed, I pulled the blanket trying to cover myself up. I was wearing a transparent black camisole decorated with sequins. I felt anxious, exposed, and I wanted to cover myself. I woke up full of panic. I was seized by a frightening tachycardia.

A few minutes passed, and she said that she felt 'numb', and then she added 'lonely'.

There was a long silence. I knew that tachycardia for my patient meant that in the next beat her heart would break. She woke up, I thought, fearing her death. This time however, I also had the explicit and clear thought that the fast heartbeat was the somatic sign of erotic feelings, pointing to the broken heart of unreciprocated love.

I sensed the anxiety in the room and in my countertransference a need to let Jasmine know that I had not left her on her own. I also had the idea of somehow communicating to her that I was not anxiously excited by her wish for me to look and touch her body.

I then decided to break the silence and I said:

A: 'In the dream you wanted to cover yourself but also you were wearing something revealing. It seems to me you dreamt of yourself caught at the crossroads of two urgent opposing needs, and that made you very anxious'.

J: [Responded quickly]: 'I could have attracted desirous looks. I was wearing something to attract'. [Pause]

A: 'K. was asleep, you thought; he would not look'.

J: 'I got very worried. I am anxious now as you are talking'.

A: 'Anxious that erotic feelings have been stirred up and that they are not going to be responded to'.

She remained silent for a while. Then she recounted an incident with her cousin. He was around eleven years old, a very good-looking boy, she admired him, she reminded me. He had demanded to see her body naked, to see her genitals. She went along with his wish. He satisfied his curiosity about her female anatomy and left. 'It was traumatic' she said. 'What seems to have been traumatic', I said, 'was not only the unboundaried coercion that you experienced and in that sense the violation of your body, but also, and maybe even more so, the possibly that it stirred up sexual feelings of your own, which you were too young to comprehend and bear'. She replied: 'The humiliation'.

After a pause I said it might be that, first and foremost, the humiliation she experienced in that encounter had to do with her not having felt desired: her body was looked at, underwent a close and detailed examination, and after that she was left, untouched, uninvited, unwanted.

There was a long silence.

My mind went back to the silence that followed my interpretation at the end of Monday's session when I talked about her wanting me to look at her breast with desire. I tried to remember the previous day's session, but nothing came to mind except her terror and agony. I thought that my commenting on her erotic feelings in the transference had psychically alarmed her, as if something traumatic had been evoked and she got 'ill' for two days.

Her words 'the humiliation' just before the present silence came back to me. It served as a link in my mind. I had the thought that the feeling of humiliation, which emerged through the analysis of the dream, was the echo from current and past experiences in and out of analysis. The humiliation of the young girl who gives in to her cousin's request to 'uncover' herself for him and feels helpless in the face of the coercion, but also the excitement brought about by this request. The girl embracing her developing pubescent body in the presence of her mother who, I had heard over the years, could not offer physical affection; she only could pat her daughter on the head at times when she wanted to express tenderness. The humiliation she had felt, without being consciously aware of it, in her current intimate and exciting, but frustrating liaison with Mr K, and the humiliation brought about by the erotic feelings in the transference. I thought that all these psychic experiences were present and reverberating, intensifying the erotic transference in the session at that moment into an unbearable feeling.

I was still feeling sad and a sense of futility when the image of a baby at the mother's breast, after the feed, and the sense of the baby's satisfaction, came into my mind. To my astonishment I felt a strong dislike for the image. I was taken aback by the strength of my reaction. Having noticed the intensity of my 'strange' response, the enacting quality of which had yet to be deciphered, allowed me to say: 'I have become the analyst/mother who does not respond to you and your body with pleasure and desire, but instead I keep my eyes shut'.

This was followed by a brief silence and then, before the end of the session, she went back to the dream. She described the image again with an almost nostalgic feeling; she described again the black camisole she was wearing, the detail of the embroidery, and she specified that it was her 'chest' that she wanted to cover 'in case he opened his eyes'.

There were a few silent moments before the end of the session.

I thought that the dream had provided us with the missing link to the split-off threatening experience borne out of the baby's struggle to tolerate the awakening of instinctual life, at a time when the yearning for sensual physical contact was not responded to in a way that would allow a sense of wellbeing. On the contrary, that very early experience, it seemed to me, had a traumatic effect.

Once dreamt and analysed, the message in the dream took its place in the chain of associations and initiated the process of restoring the representations of psychic events. I felt that in that session we had encountered a core thread in the fabric of the traumatic sense of helplessness experienced in the throes of the awakening of instinctual life.

During the period of the analysis described above, the unfolding of the somatisation proceeded from the coming into being of a transference of an eroticised need for physical closeness to the analyst; albeit, a need which had not fully emerged in the transference as yet. Furthermore, this lack of full emergence in the transference, together with the failure of the eroticised need to find fulfilment in the external object (Mr K), might well have been at the root of the return of the drive force attached to it, back to its origins in the soma.

In that first transformative moment, and under the sway of the coming into being of this transferential force, the split-off early traumatic experiences returned to be worked through. In that first instance, as there were no words for them, these experiences were 'spoken of' in the language of the body. The second moment of transformation came after the plea of the traumatic experience in the area of physical contact with the mother; it came into being through the evocation of the countertransference experience described above. With time, the transference in all its intensity was further revealed.

Following the session discussed above, we gradually became able to revisit Jasmine's symptoms: she filled her ears with 'loud noise' in order to block out the voice of what she felt to be a dangerous seduction: a love that was, as she was finding out, not reciprocated. To turn off the 'loud noise' she was hearing in the transference, she turned to illnesses: the tinnitus, on the one hand, and the tachycardia, a somatic sign itself of being in love, on the other.

Furthermore, we were able to consider the meaning of the cysts: the cysts were 'meant' to make all of us look at, think of, and touch her breast. It was the surfacing of this desire, which, in the dream, brought about tachycardia. The symptom that, as we saw, together with the tinnitus, initiated the somatisation. In the months that followed it became possible for us to reach – or rather to return – to a place where work in the preconscious and the representational field was once again possible.

In that period, we revisited the opening gesture in Jasmine's analysis. More than twenty years ago Jasmine had left the family home to pursue her studies in another part of the country. Within a month, her mother fell ill with a gastrointestinal ailment of sudden onset which unexpectedly, after only a short period of time, led to her premature death. Between the mother and the daughter, separation heralded death. Our parting, between the initial consultation and the beginning of the analysis, had psychically evoked the fear of cessation of life and led to the 'lethal pain' on the eve of the first session. In retrospect, we could think that at the moment that Jasmine was about to acquire a mother/analyst she became, at an unconscious level, terrified of experiencing separation which, for her, brings life to an end – an eventuality which casted its shadow from the dawn of our coming together.

At another level, her acting-in the body on the eve of the analysis was in later years also understood to be a warning of the dread of 'exposure' that was anticipated in analysis. The intensity of this fear was testimony of the fragility of her narcissistic equilibrium: a fragility which was revisited, time and again, and it was often announced through hypochondriacal eruptions: these were times when I was telling that her body was becoming her sole object.

Clinical case: Cate

Fotis Bobos

First initial interview with Cate

A female voice left a message on my answer phone that morning. She spoke quickly, asked if I could see her 'briefly', and concluded by saying that I had been recommended to her by a colleague, Dr D. Her request for a 'brief' visit and the rapidity of her speech annoyed me. This negative countertransferential mood was accompanied by the fantasy that the patient was not interested in long-term psychoanalytic treatment, which is what I would have preferred.

The part of her message that included her name was inaudible, and it was not possible to distinguish her first name from her surname; in fact, one of the two sounded like a male first name. This confusion about the names led to further exasperation on my part. When I rang her back, the patient clarified that it was her first name that sounded masculine, a fact which is rather unusual for Greek names.

My own countertransference towards the patient actually preceded her transference towards me. Moreover, I was a little intrigued by the idea of investigating the patient's sexual identity, given that her name sounded masculine. Five minutes after she was supposed to have arrived for her first interview, she called to complain that she had arrived at the right address, but the door had been shut, and that she was still in the vicinity and could return. In actual fact, I had not answered the door at the prearranged time. This could have been due either to my countertransference – I was too engaged in my reading to hear the doorbell – or to her own feelings of transference, which had prevented her from ringing the doorbell. In any case, there seem to have been elements of concordant countertransference along with transference. This incident shaped the beginning of our first meeting, not to mention the rest of our sessions.

The first time I saw Cate, I became perturbed. She was a tall, young woman with a scarf covering her head. The thought that she might be undergoing chemotherapy disturbed me. This image of her wearing a scarf increased my negative countertransferential feelings, but at the same time it provided me with the incentive I needed to adopt a more active attitude, one far removed from my usual psychoanalytic neutrality. Upon entering the consulting room, the patient said angrily: 'Earlier I found the door closed, but now it is open. I thought to myself, this couldn't be happening to me on top of everything else that I have to suffer! I don't even know where to begin!'

Cate went on to explain that she was forty-five, had a fifteen-year-old son, and that she was in a relationship 'that hasn't existed for a year and a half'. Moreover, she had felt 'something hard' in her breast at the beginning of the previous summer. It turned out to be cancer and she'd had twenty lymph glands removed. She concluded sardonically, 'That was the cherry on the cake. I'm now having chemotherapy'.

'Cherry on the cake?', I asked. 'Are you saying that the cake represents the relationship that doesn't exist anymore, and that the cherry stands for your breast cancer?' Here I proposed a link between the presence of a physical symptom (i.e. cancer), and the relationship that did not exist in Cate's psychic reality.

The psychoanalyst who was treating Cate's sister-in-law at the time and who had also recommended me to Cate had told her that I was very busy. This led the patient to conclude that I would not have much time for her. There were clear similarities between her idea of a non-existent relationship with her partner and her feelings of our own emerging relationship, her fantasy that I would not be able to help her, given the incident with the door.

Cate went on to say that she had always faced difficulties in her relationships 'with men, women, and everyone in general', and attributed this fact to her own 'childish' behaviour. She then became withdrawn and silent for a while before she cried: 'I'm thawing . . . Recently I have felt frozen . . . as if my life is a straight line and has no meaning'. Then she burst into sobs, and rather hesitantly took a tissue from the table.

'In all my relationships, I look for the empty spaces in the other and hasten to fill them in and meet their needs . . . and thus I lose myself. My relationships with men only last two-and-a-half years each, and then I walk away. I don't walk away entirely . . . nor do I stay', she explained.

She then expressed concern that she might use up all of my tissues. In terms of transference, she feared that by using something that belonged to me (i.e. the tissues) she might spoil or destroy me; that she would render me empty too.

Was she, perhaps, afraid that I would not give her more tissues or more time or that I wouldn't be available for her? With this in mind, I responded: 'I am not going to run out of tissues. I have more to give you'. My aim was to differentiate myself from an abandoning object.

Sobbing, Cate began to talk about her problems with her mother: '*I* got no love from her, but she loved my brother enormously. She was devoted to him, but I never got any caresses'. Cate lived alone with her son and felt lonely; this fact seems to be linked to a fundamental ambivalence that characterised her: 'I don't ask for anything, or rather, I ask a lot'. As an example of this ambivalence, she mentioned her experience of group psychotherapy two years before. She had attended sessions for two years before she was asked to leave, on the grounds that she was no longer in need of therapy. Moreover, as the oldest group member, she had adopted an advisory role towards the new members.

As she offered this information, I noticed her rocking her body back and forth while rubbing her hands at the same time; an image evocative of masturbation. This I saw as the physical manifestation of her anxiety. She then volunteered that she also had a slight problem with alcohol, as she went out drinking on her own. Or at least she used to before she started chemotherapy, but she was concerned she might relapse.

Cate used to work for her husband but since her divorce she worked as an estate agent and made a lot of money in that capacity. However, the Greek recession had made 'everything awful. I can't take it any longer; that's why I've decided to get help'. She then recalled again that Dr D had told her that I might not be available.

'What's this for?' she exclaimed suddenly, pointing at the couch. 'Do you lay people here?' At this precise moment, which was a moment of great fear for her, we heard the sound of a donkey braying nearby. Astounded at the sound, Cate asked if it was a donkey, and I confirmed that there was, indeed, a donkey in a nearby plot of land. This incident reminded her of the fact that a family of gypsies had recently come to live near her, and that this made her want to move house. In her bewilderment, she moved from the subject of 'leaving her own flat' to 'leaving her partner'. This was indicative of a fantasy that her partner might be a gypsy and it made me wonder whether, unconsciously, she feared I might be a gypsy too; that I might ask her to give me things or steal from her; that I might have too many children, that is, too many patients to have any time for her. A gypsy who wants to 'lay her on the couch', given that gypsies are often associated with a type of unrestrained sexuality that knows no bounds.

Having moved on to the subject of her partner, Cate explained that she had been with him for three or four years and that she felt as if she was 'hanging by a thread'. She was not difficult or tiresome in her relationships and she went out to bars at night. She was cool and amusing on the outside, but in turmoil on the inside. 'I'm boiling up', she sighed. 'I can hear you boiling with emotion', I offered. 'It's because no one understands me', she explained.

Cate took on a sad look and her body became still as a manifestation of her awareness of the severity of her illness. She explained that she needed to complete another course of chemotherapy before it could be decided whether a mastectomy was necessary. And if the cancer turned out to be fatal, she would not allow herself to suffer. She would commit suicide.

Somehow, she associated this idea with her mother, who claimed that her daughter's illness was not serious and that it would soon go away. 'My mother didn't know I existed', she complained. But while her sisters would run into her mother's arms as if begging her love, Cate would 'stand still': 'I would do nothing. As she paid no attention to me, I have crossed her out. When somebody doesn't listen to me, I cross them out'.

The realisation of the seriousness of her condition caused Cate to feel sad at first and then suicidal. The pain that she felt as a result of realising the severity of her physical illness and that it could lead to her death, caused her to feel great sadness and contemplate suicide as a solution. Although the thought of suicide amounts to a representation of death as a final solution, the whole process demonstrates a mental movement of narcissistic reinvestment.

Feeling that she did not really exist, as far as her mother was concerned, Cate first identified with her mother and then proceeded to eliminate her intrapsychically.

This brought me back to the door incident. I reminded Cate that she had walked away, temporarily deleting me, when I had failed to answer the door, but that she had eventually returned. Cate emphasised that she had, indeed, come back because she could not help but wonder whether she had pressed the bell long enough and whether I had forgotten about our meeting. And it was only because this thought occurred to her before she was too far away from the building, that she returned.

She then went on to talk about her family, about whom she used to talk incessantly in group therapy. Her home life had consisted of two camps: the one comprised of her and her father and the other of her mother and brother. Her sisters sat on the fence begging both for hugs and caresses. Her father could not stand her mother and was often away on business in the provinces.

Cate explained that as a child she was constantly trying to attract attention to herself. At school she used to answer back and got suspended regularly; and as an adolescent, her only interest was in boys. 'You probably think I'm childish and immature, but I have to tell you all this to get it all out', she cried. I responded by offering an interpretation of her feelings: 'So you imagine that I, just like you, consider you and your actions childish and immature and that I will also reject you'. Cate realised that she was only hurting herself by behaving in this way. 'I enjoy neither extreme', she bemoaned. 'I wish I were somewhere in the middle'.

She then moved on to the subject of ageing and the physical changes that accompany it. Her youthful appearance had always been her strong point but now her youth was abandoning her and wrinkles had started to appear. The medication she was on had caused her to gain weight. But her body had started to change before she was put on medication, she explained. Cate's sexuality used to be a central force in her behaviour. It looked as if Cate, in her outward behaviour, used her sexuality defensively via a process of overinvestment, a fact which indicates a kind of pseudo-hysterical, psychic functioning; this neurotic structure, however, was currently collapsing, thereby bringing forth her narcissistic deficits and primary psychic traumas.

In an atmosphere of emotional disappointment, the patient went on to talk about her relationship with her son, which had also changed. He was now a teenager and did not talk to her like he used to. They used to go out together, to the funfair or the cinema, but this did not happen anymore. Her son was becoming independent.

When I asked her if she dreamt, she replied that she was afraid of dreaming. She recalled a dream in which she was looking for her partner but could not find him and panicked. Then she remembered a previous dream in which she was in an art gallery admiring the paintings when, suddenly, they all disappeared.

Abruptly, Cate switched to the subject of how she was feeling. She was glad she had come to see me. The next day she was having her fifth chemotherapy treatment using a new preparation which might have side effects. Cate went on to compare the physical side effects of chemotherapy to the physical symptoms of child birth: 'At first I suffered from nausea, exhaustion and vomiting, symptoms I didn't even have during childbirth'. But now the only remaining symptom was some swelling.

All invaded tissue had been excised from the affected lymph glands and an 'in situ' tumour had been removed. When the chemotherapy treatment had been completed, the specialists would re-evaluate the situation and come to a decision with regard to whether a double mastectomy was required.

At the conclusion of the interview, I suggested we meet again at the same time in the evening, the following week. Cate responded positively to my suggestion, adding: 'I always function better at night'.

Second initial interview, a week later

'Back to my cosy nest', Cate exclaimed before settling herself in my armchair. This spontaneous formulation points to the presence of a narcissistic type of connection with me. Since our first interview, continued Cate, she had suffered from physical pain, a feeling of emptiness and depression, and had spent most of her time in bed. In the same breath she declared that she wanted to leave her partner who she saw as 'an enormous burden'. She had rejected his caresses the previous day because they gave her no satisfaction, Cate explained, and went on to rage against him for being withdrawn and unhygienic.

Her rage seemed to 'warm up' her 'frozen' body and inner world and so Cate took off her jacket and moved on to the subject of her mother who had always infuriated her. She had never been happy with her because she was too attached to her older brother and this 'got on' her 'nerves'. Her brother was all her mother had ever cared about but Cate had always had a good relationship with him and she was good friends with his wife. In fact, it was his wife who gave Cate my phone number.

'Friends? I have always had problems with my relationships. I have never had true friends', exclaimed Cate as she began to rock her body rhythmically. Even a friendly touch on the arm or leg from a girlfriend made her freeze, Cate declared. She did not believe in love and she derided any talk of love because she thought she was being used. In fact, she had never asked for caresses and hugs; she had always been 'cold and unmoved'. Her mother 'gave everything' to her brother 'but nothing' to her.

I pointed out the paradoxical similarities between Cate and her mother. The daughter asked for nothing, her mother gave her nothing. Cate agreed and added that they were also both quite 'scattered'. Her mother was involved in all sorts of social events and charities, she offered as an explanation.

At this point Cate's voice acquired a sad tone and she began to speak slower. She said that it was in our previous session that she realised the gravity of her situation. She hadn't taken it seriously before then, especially since her family and friends believed it would 'all soon go away'.

She then remembered that she had had a dream, one 'custom-made' for our session: Cate was spending the evening with one of the few female friends she possessed, Ira. Once her friend had accepted Cate's sexual advances, it transpired that Ira was actually a man. Cate admitted being at a loss as to how to interpret this particular dream; a fact that bemused her given that she was normally very good at this sort of thing: 'I analyse everything'.

I perceived that her saying the dream was 'custom-made' for me was an offer intended to fill my own void, fulfil my own desire. This might point to a repetition of her inclination to fill the void of the other. At the same time, her claim that she can 'analyse everything' might be the manifestation of a fantasy of omnipotence; a fantasy possibly projected onto me (i.e., I also analyse everything).

I decided not to comment on the dream given that its overt sexual content pointed to poor dream-work. Moreover, discussion of the patient's dreams in our first interview had indicated the presence of representational deficits attended by panic. However, it is possible that my lack of comment might have been misinterpreted as a rejection of her offer.

'I am spoilt; that's why this has happened to me!', she burst out suddenly. As evidence for this claim she cited her misbehaviour as a young girl, which was clearly designed to attract her mother's attention. 'You think you got cancer as a punishment for being spoilt?', I asked in an attempt to elaborate on the fantasy that her cancer may represent a punishment for the type of relationship she enjoyed with her mother.

Cate went on to elaborate on her childhood misdeeds, all of which had been intended to attract her mother's attention. She used to break things. At primary school she got told off a lot and was eventually expelled for circulating a diary in which Cate and her friends wrote about the boys they fancied. She had been caught red-handed. 'They destroyed me! Was what I did, really, such a terrible thing to do?', she wondered.

In an attempt to establish how her psychic life might be connected to the onset of cancer, I inquired into the events that preceded it. Although she had a lot of work, she was not making much money. She had lost her energy and was 'stuck'; 'something had to give'. She wanted her partner to move in with her, but he was not interested. She became withdrawn and felt no inclination to do anything.

'I am useless, I do nothing!', she complained as she moved on to the subject of her adolescent son wanting to leave home and move in with his father because he didn't seem to need his mother anymore. However, he had used the money he had been given the last Christmas to buy her a present, and that had really moved her. Her own mother never gave her anything and so she had 'deleted' her. I responded to this by suggesting that the feeling of emptiness she had mentioned at the beginning of our interview might be a result of her 'deleting' her mother.

At this Cate started sobbing: 'You have touched me with what you just said. You make me want to cry. This reminds me of my father'. Somehow this brought up a childhood memory according to which, once, when she was still at primary school, her father left to go on a business trip without saying goodbye to her. She had remained 'rooted to the spot' until he came back.

I was astonished to find that the association between the deficit in the mother and the void experienced by the patient should bring forth such intense emotional discharge along with a childhood memory of her father's departure. It seems to me that the father functioned as a substitute for the mother. It could also be that, in terms of massive transference, the fact that the interview was coming to an end might have contributed to the revival of a memory of depression caused by the loss of the object.

It looks as if the new circumstances of her life, namely her reduced income, her son's growing independence, her unsatisfactory relationship, and finally the new body image that comes with growing older, have had a twofold effect on her way of life. On the one hand they have imposed restrictions both on those activities that could serve as a medium through which to discharge pent-up emotion and on her previously proactive outlook towards external objects. On the other hand, her passivity and withdrawal had encouraged the self-destructive fantasy that she is useless and worth 'nothing'.

We had reached the end of the interview. I suggested meeting in a week and she agreed. Cate got up and looked around in search of a wastepaper basket. While collecting the used tissues she said: 'I'll throw these away so as not to create a mess in here'.

Thus, we embarked on a twice-weekly, face-to-face course of psychoanalytic treatment.

Sessions during her third year in psychotherapy

Cate began the session declaring that she realised that she distorts reality. The night before, she had happily tended her garden plants as if they were her own children for six whole hours before she started feeling lonely and desiring to get in touch with her partner. She wondered whether he might be with another woman, having rejected and abandoned her. She started crying. Then she called him and while they were speaking on the phone it struck her that he was a withdrawn and solitary man, and that she could not go on with him. Nevertheless, she spoke to him of her illness, explaining that a certain problem had recurred because of exposure to the sun. She then called another friend to invite him to a flamenco performance for which she had tickets. This friend had not called her in a long time and the thought that he had probably rejected her made her cry. When he spoke to her, however, he explained that he had been busy sorting out problems of his own and his telephone absence had nothing to do with her. Cate had to admit that this friend probably did still like her, and she was glad she had called him because it had helped her 'discover the truth' about him.

At this point I suggested to her that she had probably called *me* a week before my summer holiday ended for the same reason, that is, in order to find out if I was available to see her. This annoyed Cate who saw my remark as an irrelevant aside: 'You always manage to twist things and bring the subject back to our relationship. What we are doing here is different; our relationship is not one of friendship'. I pointed out that there were differences and similarities between our relationship and that of friendship and I reminded her that in a previous session she thought I wanted it to end soon so I could send her away. After this, Cate remained silent for five minutes, which I considered rather unusual. She then went on to explain that she is nothing but dull as a friend. She is actually quite amusing, but from time to time she becomes possessed by the idea that people may not like her. And this includes everyone, from schoolteachers and aunts to her own parents. Strangely enough, this idea did not occur to her the other day when she was visiting an aunt, she offered as an afterthought.

Suddenly her mood changed again, and she said angrily: 'But there are lots of asses out there, such as a certain friend of mine who throws her rubbish in my face . . . (In Greek the word 'ass' [i.e., 'donkey'] means 'rude, unsophisticated and bad-mannered'). *She* certainly doesn't like me!' I think the use of the word 'ass' is linked to the first interview. The moment she expressed the fear that I might lay her on the analyst's couch she heard a donkey braying. Perhaps through this random, perceptual, auditory cue she conceived me as a donkey that would throw her on the couch as if she were a piece of rubbish. In the same angry tone, Cate raged against her brother who was nowhere to be found while she and her sisters were trying to organise their parents' anniversary party.

Cate then resumed the subject of feeling rejected. She wondered whether her mother had wanted her to be a boy. Indeed, she had asked her mother this question once; her mother's reply had been negative, but Cate still wondered whether her mother had wanted 'a pair'. Apparently, Cate's mother had got on well with her own father but not her mother. 'But I mustn't think this way! I must reject the thought when it occurs to me. She had her reasons'. And 'maybe *you* have *your* reasons for feeling rejected', I said. 'Surely you don't mean I *need* to feel rejected?' she retorted. 'But this stops me from getting on with my life, from getting a job! I would have liked to have become a teacher even if the pay was poor. I doted on my father, but I never desired a hug from my mother'.

The very next session

The session started with Cate saying that on the way to the session she had been very concerned that she might be visited by negative thoughts again. 'Are you also concerned that I might be negative towards you?', I asked. Cate reflected on this for a little while. Then she informed me that she'd had a few dreams we could discuss, but first she would like me to know that she was having trouble sleeping because she had given up smoking pot before going to bed. She only slept in the morning for a couple of hours, after her son, Nick, left for school.

She then recounted one of the dreams: 'I lay in bed and everything around me was white; the walls, the bed, and the sheets. I felt a hand pressing down on the back of my head. I thought to myself, 'don't panic, it's only your guardian angel'. Then the pressure became a caress and my body started to float upwards . . . Once again, I thought to myself, 'don't panic, it's your guardian angel'. My nose touched the ceiling and then my body began its descent . . . I felt the hand caressing my hair, and the dream ended'.

Her next dream, she said, was about me. She dreamt that we were in my consulting room 'sleeping the whole time'. We did not talk, we just sat 'loosely' in the armchairs. I informed her, 'as always', that the session was over . . . We walked out into a large room with lots of people and a table. As we were saying our goodbyes, I kissed her on both cheeks and she asked, 'How come you kissed me on the cheeks?' I said nothing. 'Just like every other time so far', I told her that we would continue our conversation in the next session.

Having finished the narration of the dream, Cate began to remove her sweatshirt saying she was feeling hot. She explained that she had dressed warm to make sure she would not catch a cold. She then remembered that I'd had a cold the previous week and suggested I should look after myself because if I fell ill, I would be able to see neither her nor the rest of my patients.

'But what of my dream?' Cate went on. 'Is it a preparation for death? Will I die dressed in white and be resurrected into Heaven? The idea stresses me out, I don't like having to wait for it to happen'.

'You seem to be constantly afraid that something bad will happen', I said, 'and maybe you have trouble sleeping because you fear that you might have a bad dream'. 'Maybe it's because of my hormones', she said in response, 'although I've always had trouble sleeping. I've always wanted to go out and enjoy myself instead, to experience living'. I suggested that maybe she stayed up to fulfil her role as her son's guardian angel; after all, she did fall asleep and indeed dream, after her son left for school in the morning. At night, she replied, she shut all the windows in order to protect their 'nest' against anyone who might try to enter. But when she *was* able to sleep, she had no such worries, she was not concerned that someone else might come in. I used this as an opportunity to compare and contrast her trouble sleeping with the dream in which both analyst and patient remained asleep during the whole session.

After a long pause, Cate resumed the topic of her mother. She believed her mother always spoiled everything, and so she was afraid that her mother might also spoil the party for her fiftieth wedding anniversary. But Cate had come to realise that *she* also spoiled everything because she was her mother's daughter in this respect.

Nevertheless, Cate tried to encourage her mother to think positively so as not to spoil the party. She also tried to boost the morale of her partner who sounded depressed on the phone. But she did not visit him; she was able to control herself. She knew that if she had gone to see him, they would have had sex and she did not want that to happen.

Next, I discussed the connection between her attempt to encourage her mother and cheer up her partner, and the dream in which her body rose up to the ceiling. This image of her body floating upwards, I interpreted as an indication that she was already feeling 'uplifted'.

Cate responded by saying that if she was uplifting others, then she was probably uplifted herself. She realised that she needed to stop inventing scenarios which conclude in her being rejected by other people. This was exactly what her ex-husband George did. He kept inventing scenarios and theories to explain other people's behaviour. For example, he had come to the conclusion that their son, Nick, was considering seeing a psychotherapist because he felt rejected. Cate recommended that they both stopped theorising and started minding their own business. 'We still have a long way to go', she concluded.

References

Aisenstein, M. (2006) 'The indissociable unity of psyche and soma: a view from the Paris Psychosomatic School', *Int. J. Psychoanal.*, 87, pp. 667–80.

Racker, H. (1957) 'The meaning and uses of countertransference', *Psychoanalytic Quarterly*, 26, pp. 303–57.

Section II

Clinical pictures

Chapter 1

Depression and psychosomatics

JACQUES PRESS

Depression in psychosomatics cannot be tackled without referring to the notion of essential depression. Developed by Pierre Marty, this notion indeed holds a pivotal place in Marty's theoretical model, as well as in the subsequent work of the Paris Psychosomatic School. I will therefore begin with a recapitulation of some of its basic elements and will then question its limitations on the basis of the clinical cases presented in this volume. More specifically, I will stress the medical and objectifying dimension of Marty's notion, which led him to overlook a few key countertransferential issues. I will then expound a personal perspective on depression and psychosomatics, with an emphasis on the importance of Winnicott's notion of fear of breakdown and on the dynamics of flight that it entails, which also connect to the play of transference and countertransference.

Essential depression in classical psychosomatic theory

Working in somatic hospitals, the psychosomatic therapists of the Paris School were struck by a particular form of mental functioning which they encountered in some of their patients. These individuals expressed no demand for psychological support, which was understandable: they were physically ill and preoccupied with their illness. But a striking feature was that they showed no interest in their psychic life. Relatedly, their mode of thinking was concrete and limited to an affectless account of daily life events without any discernible fantasmatic activity in the background. This state of affairs led Marty and his colleagues to the well-known concept of operative thinking – a concept that has been the victim of its own success and used in ways that are improper and often operative in itself, like a recipe likely to yield an easy diagnosis. Subsequently, Marty coined the term 'operative life' to underline the fact that such modality of functioning not only pertained to thinking but in fact pervaded the whole life of these individuals.

Yet, interestingly, many of these patients did not always have this presentation. Their family and friends, and sometimes the patients themselves, would remember times when they were more alive, but also more difficult to live with due to their temperamental traits. Such traits seemingly faded without a trace, as if they had undergone some kind of silent abrasion. From this observation stems Marty's insistence on the importance of the psychosomatic investigation (see Chapter 4, 'Psychosomatic investigation and treatment'), which is endowed with a double aim: eliciting a return to the traumatic factors that might have led to this gradual process of psychic extinction and understanding the path that such a process took. The investigation therefore aims to foreground the differences between the current functioning (now) and the usual functioning (prior to the disorganisation resulting in the present illness).

For Marty, it became clear that this path took on a distinct depressive modality, which he referred to as essential depression: a form of depression precisely characterised by a robotisation and an impoverishment of mental functioning – by the operative life I just mentioned, in other words. The two terms – operative life and essential depression – are therefore two sides of the same coin; they account for two complementary aspects of the same phenomenon of psychic impoverishment, which must always be gauged dynamically.

Let us take anxiety, for example. Characteristically, massive and generally diffuse forms of anxiety can be found in many of these patients, as is the case with Cate, Fotis Bobos's patient. The reduction, if not the disappearance, of such anxieties can follow from two distinct and conflicting processes: either the patient gets better and returns to his or her former functioning, or conversely, essential depression progresses relentlessly, and the patient's instinctual life becomes so impoverished that the patient loses the ability to mobilise any anxious reaction. Reciprocally, the worsening of anxiety can result from the same two conflicting movements. With reorganisation, the anxieties that had disappeared resurface because, psychically speaking, the patient is coming back to life. With disorganisation, for an individual who formerly did not present any anxieties or only anxieties of an objectal kind, diffuse anxieties emerge owing to the breakdown of psychic defences, as evident in the case of Jasmine, Marina's patient.

Gauging the severity and the dynamics of essential depression is therefore a central issue in the psychosomatic investigation, all the more so as, in Marty's view, this form of depression leads to death more surely than does melancholia itself.

Countertransferential issues and flight before the fear of breakdown

Such is the 'classical' theory developed by Pierre Marty in the 1960–1980 period (Marty, 1976, 1980). What have we learned since then and to what extent do Marty's basic assumptions remain relevant? Two questions arise. First of all, while essential depression doubtlessly exists, can we posit with certainty that it should be involved in all processes of disorganisation? Could there be other paths leading to somatic illness? The second issue lies in the fact that the notions of essential depression and operative life are so tightly enmeshed in Marty's theoretical presuppositions that their use becomes difficult if we do not endorse them wholly. More specifically, as I argued elsewhere, Marty's position is a medical one that envisions the patient in an objectifying way (Press, 2016). As a result, he not only tends to overlook a few pivotal countertransferential issues at play with psychosomatic patients, he also displays countertransference resistance through his theorising process itself. This is the case when, for example, Marty describes his patients as 'incomplete' before an analyst who would conversely be 'complete' because he or she has reached an optimal – i.e. oedipal – level of functioning. Due to these limits, I am urged to reformulate Marty's central intuition in my own terms.

Let us take Cate, Fotis's patient, as the starting point of my reflection. Her case is especially illustrative indeed. Cate undoubtedly presents a depressive state with little guilt, and an accumulation of traumatic factors culminating in the discovery of her cancer. However, I would refrain from appending the term 'essential depression' to her, as such a diagnosis might reduce her to a clinical 'case' used to corroborate Marty's theory. I am much more interested in the first contingencies of her meeting with her analyst, a meeting that almost did not take place due to the problems with the doorbell. Did Cate not ring the bell, or did Fotis fail to hear her? The question remains open and is ultimately rather unimportant. Highly significant, conversely, is the fact that this nearly missed encounter exposes a key element in the patient's psychic construction – the impossible encounter with her mother which pervades the first two sessions of investigation. Her 'solution' consisted in cutting her mother off, and in so doing cutting off an important part of herself, as Fotis rightfully points out. But in my view, one must take into account the fact that the non-meeting with the object comes first while the patient's 'solution', however costly it may be, consists in an attempt to annul or erase the primary and essential wound.

The problem lies in the psychic and psychosomatic cost of the means mobilised in order to reach this goal. In Bionian terms, we could say that Cate chooses the evacuation over the metabolisation of frustration (Bion, 1962, pp. 30–34). Or, as Winnicott would put it, she is constantly 'flying into sanity' (Winnicott, 1954, p. 287) in a kind of disorganised hyperactivity akin to manic defence, with a view to avoiding the experience of 'unthinkable agony' (Winnicott, 1965, p. 127), of breakdown (Winnicott, 1974). Over the years, I have come to think that many of these patients might become physically ill when this 'flight into sanity' reaches its limits, either out of exhaustion or due to external events. The somatic illness could somehow arise in lieu of a breakdown (Press, 2016). This outlook has proven more helpful to me in terms of understanding my patients than a reference to essential depression. It forces us to step out of a diagnostic approach and to make the fear of breakdown and the dynamics of flight that it entails the central stake in the play of transference and countertransference in these situations.

Along the same lines, the dreams recounted by the patient during the investigation are extremely significant. During the initial session, she recounts two. In the first one, 'she was looking for her boyfriend and she couldn't find him, she was panicked'. I am inclined to think that lurking behind the friend is the figure of the mother, and that this dream is about the impossible encounter with the latter. This naturally does not imply that more elaborate erotic and aggressive impulses should not be operative and worthy of analysis, but the fundamental problem lies elsewhere. In the second dream, 'she was in an art gallery watching the paintings. Suddenly all of them disappeared'. This is a prime example of negative hallucination. But, once again, the process of negativation seems to actively repeat, in my view, something that was first experienced passively, i.e. the non-meeting with the object. The contrast with the dream recounted during the second session of investigation is all the more significant. Cate established an early transference of an intensely positive nature, coming to her session as if it were her 'cosy nest'. She then recounts a dream in which she approaches a girlfriend with a sexual intent and this girlfriend turns out to be a man – her analyst. In other words, she is looking for a maternal figure and this maternal figure becomes embodied in the analyst. In my view, this dream is evidence of the beginning of a process of psychic reawakening: there is now an object that she can strive to reach. There is hope too, however fragile it might be. The very first sign of potential hope lies in the way Cate solved the problem with the doorbell: granted, she left but she also came back.

What were the factors leading to disorganisation in Cate's case? We have little information on the subject and are therefore bound to speculate. She might have experienced her divorce as a kind of ultimate confirmation: she was unable to sustain a loving relationship and escape her mother. The difficulties she encountered with her real estate agency, which had probably provided a vital source of narcissistic gratification, might have also had a disorganising impact on her. And the cherry on the cake was the catastrophic state of her relationship with her friend, which could have resonated with the failure of her marriage by reactualising it.

I would not want to conclude without saying a few words about Jasmine, Marina's patient. Here we have a very different picture. Jasmine seems to have achieved a much more stable and better organised level of functioning. Deep within her, a wound remains – a secret wound but a deep one all the same. It is hidden behind her 'wish to start analysis', which she initially states as self-evident. As with Cate, this wound stems from the vicissitudes of the primary narcissistic tie with the mother and it surfaces fleetingly during the sessions of investigation when she mentions the moments when life seemed futile or grey to her. At the outset, depression is seemingly not a feature of the picture; but this account is a mistake. Depression is featured; indeed, it is merely veiled and only becomes exposed in the 'grey' moments. Furthermore, the acute pain that emerges on the eve of the first session on the couch is an episode which seems to show that, short of finding a psychic outcome, the drive-related impulses at play by preference take on a somatic form of expression, alternating or coexisting with massive and diffuse anxiety.

An especially significant aspect of this case is the enmeshment of narcissistic and erotic factors, which the analytic couple eventually managed to unfurl. I will discuss this point in more detail in the chapter 'Psychosomatic investigation and treatment', so I will limit myself to one comment here. Marina's decisive interpretation – 'I have become the analyst/mother who does not respond to you and your body with pleasure and desire, but instead I keep my eyes shut' – draws its force from two elements. First of all, it brings together, within one sentence, the narcissistic and intensely erotic impulses. Secondly, the very fact that the analyst refers to herself as a mother 'with the eyes shut', means she offers herself as a highly libidinal transferential figure. This statement leads me to make an important final point. What makes breakdown a state with such serious consequences is not only the fact that the object is irremediably lost, but equally that such a loss leaves the infant exposed to some drive-related inflow, which he or she is completely unequipped to face. In the long term, this state of affairs may lead to a psychic construction in which any manifestation of the drives is experienced as a major danger. As a consequence, the only way out consists in extinguishing at the root anything akin to drive-related activity, and this wish for extinction can contribute to the risk of somatic illness.

To conclude, the notion of essential depression retains some degree of diagnostical value in my view, but it is embedded in an objectifying theoretical model which limits its application. Furthermore, clinically speaking and as is evident in Cate's case, I often find that attention to the forms of hyperactivity connoting a possible manic defence can be more useful. Even more importantly, an objectifying perspective may prevent us from tolerating and fully experiencing the countertransferential impact of the modalities of defence. The patient is hyperactive because he or she strives to flee from a threat of breakdown that goes back to early infancy, and because the patient has been unable to construct a reliable, internal object to lean upon. Such a constellation is likely to preside over the analytic situation as a whole, and pervade the transference and countertransference; it will be the responsibility of the analytic couple to experience this state of affairs with a view to eventually detangling it.

NICK TEMPLE

The concept of depression is important in a psychoanalytic understanding of psychosomatic conditions because depression represents a conflict with an internal object. This object is persecuting and dominates the superego, menacing the patient. The question at stake here is the extent to which this conflict is defended against by being displaced into the body as a somatic symptom. Some individuals seem to be predisposed to this vulnerability by their early history. Bion enlarged on the danger of an unreconstructed superego in his theory of containment; he emphasised that a failure in maternal containment results in 'an object which when installed in the patient exercises the function of a severe and ego-destructive superego' (Bion, 1959, p. 107). Britton has pointed out that this situation can lead to negative therapeutic reactions in response to the patient's progress or success in analysis (Britton, 2003).

McDougall described similar forms of failed containment in the maternal relationship in the early history of psychosomatic patients, which can lead to problems in expressing and symbolising affect (McDougall, 1989). She also helpfully reminds us that we can all be prone to somatic reactions under difficult circumstances of stress: 'Clinical observation slowly taught me that all analysands and analysts as well somatise at one time or other particularly when stressful events override their usual ways of coping with mental pain and conflict' (McDougall, 1989, p. 3).

There are two contrasting descriptions of depression in psychosomatic illness: the first is 'essential' depression where the individual is cut off from affect and the conflict is displaced into somatic symptoms. This is in contrast to the second, which might be described as 'melancholic' depression, where there is an active preoccupation with mental pain, guilt and feelings of badness that may involve suicidal thoughts. In this type of depression there is continual conflict with an internal object dominating the superego who criticises and blames the patient for being bad.

Pierre Marty, of the Paris School of Psychosomatics, describes essential depression as occurring in psychosomatic illness; he sees essential depression as a depression without pain, without an object and without guilt, in which there is a lowering of libidinal drive. Feelings of devaluation, and of having sustained a narcissistic wound, are often replaced by tiredness or over-activity, which do not contribute to self-esteem. Essential depression may precede 'mechanical life', a concept that closely resembles that of alexithymia, described by Sifneos (Sifneos, 1975, pp. 65–70). Marty's idea is that that the somatic manifestation replaces a conflicted situation. He proposes that psychosomatic illnesses act like points of fixation in a movement towards more general mental and physical disorganisation. He gives the name 'progressive disorganisation' (Marty, 1968) to the process by which there is destruction of the actual libidinal organisation in an individual. Progressive disorganisation can become an anarchic destruction of mental functions and entail a cancellation of libidinal functions that can lead to a general decathexis of all libidinal areas, producing essential depression. Organising mental function such as identification, projection, association of ideas and symbolisation disappear. This process shows how the death instinct asserts itself and can end in death through serious somatic illness (Marty, 1968).

We seem here to be dealing with a situation in which the painful depressive conflict with an internal object has been split off and located in the body, and it does not appear to be represented in the mind. In this sense, the patient might be described as substituting physical pain and disability for psychic pain, which operates as a defence in order to avoid the disturbing aspects of the conflict and affect associated with it. It could be that the dangerous nature of the internal conflict is a function of the paranoid/schizoid position, as described by Klein. The patient does not easily have the capacity to move into the depressive position and therefore cannot mourn separation or tolerate ambivalence. If this can be become part of the analytic work in the transference relationship, movement is enabled towards a more integrated state. This will be facilitated by the analyst's capacity to contain and tolerate the negative transference. Here, a consideration of the technique of working with psychosomatic patients requires some discussion. For example, in view of the possible vulnerability of psychosomatic patients to exploration of the negative transference, should work in the negative transference, which might lead to deterioration in the somatic illness, be undertaken? Bronstein (Bronstein, 2011) states that it does not altogether seem justifiable on theoretical or clinical grounds to make changes in analytical technique or avoid work in the negative transference to make the work more supportive.

Aisenstein (Aisenstein, 1993) describes a patient in a state of essential depression who was suffering from severe haemorrhagic rectocolitis. The patient is shut off from his feelings, and his emotional life and physical condition will likely lead to major surgery. Aisenstein's interpretative work with the patient brings about changes in the patient in which he begins to feel guilt and depressive pain about his first wife. At the same time, there is much improvement in his illness. The changes are first represented in a nightmare in which he sees his first wife covered in blood, and her life can only be saved by being given an artificial anus. Further analysis leads the patient to be able to mourn the loss of his first wife and accept the damage he did to her. At this point, he becomes able to have a child with his second wife. This case illustrates the patient's movement from a somatised state of essential depression with severe psychosomatic symptoms, through a melancholic guilty depressed state, to reach a more mature capacity for sadness and mourning.

Essential depression is strikingly in contrast to 'melancholic' depression (I have used this term to denote a state of depression similar to melancholia, as described by Freud in 'Mourning and Melancholia': Freud, 1917), where there are strong negative affects and experiences of guilt and badness. This type of depression represents an active and painful state, where the conflict with the internal figure is represented as a conscious fantasy involving guilty self-reproaches. These feelings are experienced painfully in the transference relationship where the analyst will be felt to become critical and judgemental. In this state, feelings of guilt and suffering arise, and these are disturbing and frightening and involve fear of damage and retaliation. In some patients, as the somatic illness improves, painful depressive feelings develop. In both Marina Perris's patient Jasmine and Fotis Bobos's patient Cate, we see depressive feelings and negative feelings towards the analyst alternating with psychosomatic symptoms. These physical symptoms represent a retreat from the painful, guilty feelings. Jasmine has abdominal pain, tinnitus, tachycardia, and hypertension. Cate has breast cancer.

These patients illustrate the complex interplay between the superego figure associated with depression on the one hand, and the somatic symptoms on the other hand. Jasmine, who is eager to start in analysis and idealises the analyst, nevertheless develops severe abdominal pain the day before her first session. Fotis's patient Cate seems to be in this persecuted state as soon as she comes to see him; she is expecting to be shutout and the problem around Fotis answering the doorbell only confirms her conviction. Before even meeting Fotis, Cate is convinced he wants to reject her. In contrast, Marina's patient Jasmine wishes to idealise her from the first meeting and to avoid the ambivalence in the relationship. When the analyst shows a capacity to explore the negative assumptions without retaliation he can then begin to be felt as more supportive and in touch with the patient's distress. This seems to have been what happened with Cate: through exploring with Fotis her perception that he was keeping her out, she was able move away from the more paranoid view of her relationship with her analyst.

Psychosomatic symptoms can develop at points of psychic change when movement in analysis causes disturbance to the internal equilibrium. This could have occurred in the case of Jasmine when she has an abdominal pain that she describes as lethal the night before her first session. Starting the analysis represents an important psychic move for her in struggling with her depressive feelings and their origins in her childhood experiences.

When patients present with psychosomatic symptoms, or develop them during the course of the analysis, it is possible that a painful and disturbing relationship with an internal figure has become located in the body as a result of projection. This can result in a defensive lack of contact with affect, leading to operational thinking or alexithymia. It is difficult to unravel the nature of the conflictful relationship being defended against, but in some clinical situations somatic symptoms may develop in reaction to interpretations in analysis. This happened with a young female patient, Sally, who developed an asthma attack following my transference interpretation of her ambivalence towards me, which suggested that her hostile thoughts had to be defended against. The emotional connections to longstanding somatic symptoms can be more difficult to establish, and can take careful analytic work to gauge, but the content of transference and countertransference can throw light on them. An example of a longstanding displacement of a painful conflict into the body was my patient Donald, a man of forty who had developed epileptic fits after the death of his mother at the age of fifteen, and he continued to have fits whenever he experienced an emotionally stressful situation. In both Donald and the asthmatic patient there was a limited capacity to be in touch with powerful affects or to experience the conflict in a direct way.

The onset of somatic symptoms might also be seen as negative therapeutic reactions to an improvement in the patient's state of mind. This might arise in analysis when significant psychic movement is occurring in an attempt to separate from a claustrophobic relationship with a primary object; the result can be an experience of anguish that separation and autonomy is a terrible disloyalty, which gives rise to guilt and depression. In one instance, Sally, the young woman described above developed asthma and allergies in her analysis after she made significant moves to separate from a guilty and persecuted internal relationship with her mother who had died during her adolescence.

When Jasmine, Marina's patient, has the dream in the Wednesday session, her internal conflict is portrayed in the transference relationship. At this point, Jasmine's ambivalent internal conflict has begun to move from her body to become symbolically represented in her mind. This indicates the development of a capacity to symbolise the conflict and to explore it in the transference, which might be seen as facilitated by the analyst's interpretative exploration. We could see this as a shift from the paranoid position, in which guilt is experienced as persecutory, towards the depressive position, where there is a greater capacity for sadness.

My patient Sally's somatic symptoms decreased as she began to have dreams which represented her guilt about her breaking free from the internal relationship and which involved her anger towards the controlling internal figure. She also experienced me, her analyst, in the transference as a rigid, judgemental figure. It was possible to explore this in the transference relationship when she took up independent positions from me, and was able to argue with strength, despite her fear that she'd caused serious damage. Part of Sally's somatic symptoms involved inflammation of her salivary gland, which led to a conviction that she was developing cancer of the throat – the disease that caused her mother's death. There appeared to be a connection between the swelling of her salivary gland and her history of chewing thread, which itself was connected to a relic of a relationship with an original transitional object, originally a blanket which had been chewed into threads. This relationship had not been resolved but remained as the compulsive habit of chewing thread. The improvement in her somatic symptoms led to a period of serious melancholic depression, in which she felt bad and guilty, and this was worked through over many months in the analysis. As a result of this analytic work, the patient was able to make progress in her career and started a successful relationship with a man whom she later married.

In my discussion of the different forms of depression in somatic states, I have considered two distinct types of depression: essential depression and melancholic depression. These two types of depression can be seen to be on a developmental continuum from a defended state in which painful conflict is displaced into somatic symptoms with avoidance of painful affect, moving towards a melancholic state of depression, in which the conflict becomes expressed and can be symbolised in dreams with the painful, guilty affect that had previously been avoided. Further development leads in the direction of more mature, sad and depressive affects in relation to the conflict. I have discussed how analytic work focused on the transference can facilitate psychic change, with movement along a continuum in the direction of more mature guilt and a greater capacity to mourn. This might possibly be represented as a movement from the paranoid position to the depressive position in Klein's terms. The patient is released from somatic symptoms and able to struggle with guilty conflicts, which takes place through a greater capacity for mourning and sadness, accompanied by more mature autonomy.

Commentary

EVA SCHMID-GLOOR

The contributions from Jacques Press and Nick Temple show interesting differences. Jacques displays a sceptical position when it comes to the value of links between depression and psychosomatics. He thinks that Marty's concept of 'essential depression' retains its value from a diagnostic point of view but has limitations in its clinical use. Jacques takes his distance from an 'objective' point of view, which for him characterises the observations in Marty's classical theory, where depression is marked by an impoverishing of mental functioning and linked with 'operative life' and the machine-like functioning of psychosomatic patients.

Jacques points out that Marty was examining the patients in a rather objective way and therefore acted from a medical position, so that he didn't take into account major issues in the countertransference. Jacques then concentrates on what we have learned since Marty and brings into discussion two main questions which he considers to be crucial. He is sure that essential depression exists, but he asks whether a traumatic situation necessarily leads to it, and whether there might be other paths leading to somatisation. He therefore reformulates Marty's intuition and distances himself from a nosological approach, which for him cuts off important aspects that he wants to focus on, in particular the crucial role of countertransference. Jacques thinks that when Marty describes his patients as 'incomplete', as having a lack in mental functioning, he is acting out his countertransference resistance in the very process of his theoretical modelling.

In his discussion of Fotis Bobos's case with the patient who presents aspects of an atypical depression, with little guilt feelings and an accumulation of traumatic factors in her life, Jacques would hesitate to qualify her depression as 'essential'. Jacques concentrates on the start of the treatment, where Fotis and the patient get caught up in a situation which shows an impossible encounter with the object. As the patient says, her solution to her problematic relation with her mother was to 'cut her mother off', and by doing so she cut off an important part of herself. As Jacques understands it, the 'cutting off' is an effort to make a fundamental and unbearable failure unreal and non-existent. The patient chooses evacuation rather than metabolisation of frustration. In Winnicottian terms, she is constantly 'flying into sanity', into a hyperactivity in order to avoid a confrontation with a state of 'unthinkable agony' and breakdown. Jacques' idea is that patients fall somatically ill, when – out of inner or outer reasons – 'flight into sanity', which still binds some drive energy, stops being possible. This idea helped Jacques on a technical level to work with his psychosomatic patients much more than did the process of looking for essential depression. We can understand what an effort must be made in countertransferential involvement and containment when it comes to the patient's catastrophising and the failure of his/her previously functioning survival mode.

For Jacques, the essence of the depression of Fotis's patient is a process of negativation in which the patient actively repeats what she had first passively gone through. The early loss might leave the child exposed to a drive overflow, and this can lead to a situation in which any drive-laden manifestation becomes a major danger, which leads the patient to suppress any libidinal motion, and so contributes to the risk of somatisation.

Nick Temple takes a very different position concerning the question of depression in psychosomatics. He confirms the crucial role which depression plays in psychosomatic illness, but he locates the source of it differently to Jacques. While Jacques understands depression to be caused by a process of negativation linked to an unbearable early experience, Nick states that depression represents the expression of a conflict with an internal object, which is finally displaced into the body. Whereas in Jacques' understanding the object relation is lost, in Nick's understanding the object is present, but it is torturing and persecuting the subject. Nick speaks of a 'persecuting object which dominates the superego and menaces the patient'. The origin of the depression for Nick is not a negativation process, but the conflict of the subject with its persecuting object that becomes a severe and ego-destructive superego.

We can see here a link with Jacques' position, where he points out that any drive-laden manifestation (which avoids repeating the early non-containment), can be experienced as menacing and therefore gets split off. But still, in Jacques' position the object is missing which delivers the subject to a drive overflow and over-excitation, whereas in Nick's position the object is present and torturing the subject by persecuting it. We might ask ourselves, whether a drive overflow, caused by the absence of the object, can be experienced as persecuting as well.

We can see here two different positions in technique. Jacques' position would ask the analyst to contain their own difficult experiences of countertransference and help the patient to integrate the unbearable and therefore negative. Nick thinks that with melancholic depression, the analyst would at first have to bear the negative transference, so that the patient could contain his/her guilt feelings and move from the paranoid position in which guilt is experienced as persecutory towards the depressive position, where there is a greater capacity for sadness and mourning.

The two authors show interesting differences, above all when it comes to technical questions. Jacques' approach is to contain and live through a breakdown with his patient, in which there is no object present. In Jacques' understanding, psychosomatic patients constantly and desperately try to flee from a breakdown; this breakdown is linked to an early traumatic experience with an absent object. Jacques would strive with his patients to live through this absence, failure and non-containment by the object, and would accept becoming this failing object for his patient. He would live through the accusations and attacks from his patients, and he would aim to survive them. For Jacques, the analyst's task would at first be to concentrate on the needs of the patient and to feel his/her pain. In a sense, Jacques' formulation of a patient who feels overwhelmed by an excess of drive flooding might link with Nick's notion of persecution, since the excess drive might also be experienced as persecuting.

When it comes to Nick, he is interested in using the transference to work through the conflict of his patient with a too rigid and cruel superego, which stems from a persecuting object. His technique would involve becoming this persecuting object for his patient, so that the object could become represented, analysed and integrated.

We can perceive in these two contributions the different theoretical positions of the authors and the very interesting dialogue that takes place. In Jacques' part, the theory of negativation is at stake: we can see a 'disobjectalising function' like that described by André Green (1993), who links drive theory with object relations theory; in Jacques' theoretical background, depression arises from the disobjectalising function – when the relationship with the object is too painful the subject decathects the object, so that the object becomes absent and the subject flees; but this also gives rise to an over-excitation which can be experienced as persecutory. As such, we are left wondering whether the 'fear of breakdown', from which Jacques' patient tries to flee, and the persecutory object, from which the patient of Nick's flees, are quite as different as one might think.

References

Aisenstein, M. (1993) 'Psychosomatic solution or somatic outcome: the man from Burma. Psychotherapy of a case of haemorrhagic rectocolitis', *Int. J. Psychoanal.*, 74, pp. 371–38.

Bion, W. (1959) *Second Thoughts*. Northvale, NJ: Jason Aronson.

Bion, W. (1962) *Learning from Experience.* New York: Basic Books.

Britton, R. (2003) *Sex, Death, and the Superego: Experiences in Psychoanalysis*. London: Karnac.

Bronstein, C. (2011) 'On Psychosomatics: The Search For Meaning', *Int. J. Psychoanal.*, 92, pp. 173–95.

Freud, S., Freud, A. and Strachey, J. (1917) 'Mourning and Melancholia', in *The Standard Edition of the Complete Psychological Works of Sigmund Freud.* London: The Hogarth Press, 1973.

Green, A. (1993) 'Pulsion de mort, narcissisme négatif, function désobjectalisante', in *Le travail du négatif.* Paris: Les Éditions de Minuit.

Marty P. (1968) 'A Major Process of Somatization: The Progressive Disorganization', *Int. J. Psychoanal.*, 49, pp. 246–49.

Marty, P. (1976) *Les mouvements individuels de vie et de mort.* Paris: Payot.

Marty, P. (1980) *L'ordre psychosomatique*. Paris: Payot.

McDougall, J. (1989) 'The body mind-matrix', in *Theatres of the Body: A Psychoanalytic Approach to Psychosomatic Illness*. London: Free Association Books.

Press, J. (2016) 'Metapsychological and clinical aspects of psychosomatics research', *Int. J. Psychoanal.*, 97, pp. 89–113.

Sifneos, P.E. (1975) 'Problems of psychotherapy with patients with alexithymia characteristics and physical disease', *Psychother Psychosom*, 26, pp. 65–70.

Winnicott D.W. (1954) 'Metapsychological and clinical aspects of regression within the psycho-analytical set-up', in *Through Paediatrics to Psycho-analysis*. London: The Hogarth Press, pp. 278–94.

Winnicott, D.W. (1965) 'The psychology of madness: a contribution from psychoanalysis', in Winnicott, D.W. (1989), *Psycho-analytic Explorations*. London: Karnac.

Winnicott D.W. (1974) *Fear of Breakdown in Psychoanalytic Explorations*. Edited by C. Winnicott, R. Shepherd and M. Davis. London: Karnac, 1989.

Chapter 2

Trauma and its effects

FOTIS BOBOS

Introduction

In his last papers, Freud focuses his attention on trauma and the mechanism of splitting. He also explores the analyst's therapeutic constructions in order to deal with traumatic 'fixations' manifesting either as a positive effect, namely a 'compulsion to repeat' the traumatic situation, or as a negative one, 'defensive reactions', both of which contribute to character formation. Freud (Freud, 1939, p. 73) refers to 'cases which are distinguished as being 'traumatic' because their effects go back unmistakably to one or more powerful impressions in these early times – impressions which have escaped being dealt with normally'.

By 'normally' Freud refers to psychic processing of external or internal excitations. He characterises as 'traumatic' those cases where an excess in demand is responsible for pathological reactions 'only as a result of a quantitative factor'. In the same text, Freud concludes that, 'The traumas are either experiences on the subject's own body or sense perceptions, mostly of something seen and heard – that is, experiences or impressions' (Freud, 1939, p. 74).

About half a century earlier, in his early drafts on hysteria, Freud (1892, p. 154) defines psychic trauma thus: 'any impression which the nervous system has difficulty in disposing of by means of associative thinking or of motor reaction becomes a psychic trauma'. In this definition of psychic trauma, he also includes the body in its motor reaction. Therefore, at the time of traumatism, Freud distinguishes the hindrances that the subject encounters in both directions – in associative thinking and in somatic discharge via motor reaction. The deficiency of the subject's reaction (psychic or motor) is the common denominator in both directions.

In the meantime, Ferenczi, as an inspiring writer who was closely interested in traumatic situations, postulates that trauma is a 'shock, that is an annihilation of self-regard – of the ability to put up a resistance, and to act and think in defence of one's own self' (Ferenczi, 1932, pp. 253–54). Furthermore, Ferenczi suggests that 'perhaps even the organs which secure self-preservation give up their function or reduce it to a minimum . . . Shock can be purely physical, purely moral, or both physical and moral'. I think that Ferenczi's definition of trauma as a moral shock, which is a sudden blow to the mind, is synonymous with Freud's definition; both authors underline the destructive effects of trauma on thinking and reacting. Nevertheless, Ferenczi goes one step further by creating a potential link between a traumatic situation and the dysfunctioning of organs, thus offering a psychosomatic perspective.

Some comparative observations and comments on the two clinical cases

I think that, by comparing the two clinical cases of Marina Perris and my own, it is particularly important to investigate the qualitative characteristics of the irregular psychosomatic organisations and functions from the perspective of the Paris Psychosomatic School. More specifically, I refer to some important features of somatic symptoms, which in each case designate the degree and extent of psychic deficiencies. According to this approach, we can distinguish schematically between two categories of somatisations: a) severe malignant somatic diseases, which are caused by the silent, chronic process of drive defusion, namely progressive disorganisation, and can lead to a subject's death; b) repetitive, benign somatisations that appear in short term relapses and arise from the mechanism of somatic regression. Somatic regression is a somatic defence mechanism that responds to a traumatic situation and constitutes a point of somatic fixation, which therefore forms a barrier against further disorganisation (Marty, 1980; Smadja, 2001).

My first observation concerning Jasmine is that the bodily symptoms arising during the analysis are involved in the relationship with the analyst, as a reactivation of early traumas. In contrast, Cate suffered from the somatic symptom before coming to the analysis and it was the main reason for seeking help. My second observation concerns the qualitative differences between the psychosomatic organisation in the two cases. Although the two patients suffer from somatic illnesses of a specific erotogenic bodily zone, namely the breast, there are significant differences in the quality of the symptoms, with obvious consequences both at the psychic and the somatic level. Jasmine suffers from several functional somatic symptoms (symptoms without tissue damage) such as acute abdominal pain, tinnitus, hypertension and tachycardia, and only later on does she develop the organic symptom (symptom with tissue damage) of benign cysts in her breast. Cate, on the somatic level, suffers from a severe life-threatening illness: breast cancer.

My third observation concerning Jasmine is that because of her functional symptoms and cysts she develops a temporary hypochondriacal defensive organisation of the type of actual neurosis (Freud, 1914, p. 83). With regard to her psychic organisation, Cate seems to suffer from 'character neurosis' traits.[1]

Cate

Cate's psychic difficulties, which were manifested mostly on a behavioural level, were encountered even before the first interview. Movements of going forwards and backwards, both on a motor and psychic level, were repetitively present during the first interviews. The quick alternations of her psychic movements from one direction to the opposite constitute a projection of the psychic instability of her inner world, as well as feelings of great anxiety. These repetitive and monotonous motor and psychic hyperactive movements are at the same time in accordance with the psychic state of being cold, unmoved, immobilised at the same point, as she emphatically describes herself.

The explosiveness of her reactions and the rapid rhythm of her speech give me the feeling of an immediate danger, a fixation on a state of helplessness. During the interviews, her volatile temper seems to depict her character traits manifesting her defensive aggressive mode of relatedness with other people. She shows herself to be extremely sensitive to perceptive stimuli from the environment (the closed door, the analyst having no vacancy for her, the couch, the donkey) in a transient, paranoid, psychic state, expressing the feeling of being threatened and rejected by the analyst. After sobbing with tears as a physical sign of sadness, she gets on to slowly talking about her relationship with her family and mostly with her mother. The feelings of disappointment and injustice pour out from every area of her life.

The reference to the 'empty spaces' projected into the other is a marker of her active psychic trauma. Early psychic trauma appears as a screen memory on the scene of the violent disputes of the opposing camps in her family: she is aligned with her father against her mother and brother. Cate rejects with aversion her younger sister who stands 'as a beggar asking for hugs and kisses', actually a representation of a repudiated part of herself. Recent changes and losses in her life seem to have operated as agents that activate traumatic zones in her unstable and fragile psychosomatic equilibrium.

Jasmine

From the first consultation, the analyst notices with Jasmine hasty, repetitive reactions of 'a sense of urgency', which she makes in order to avoid something unpleasant and unknown. In the second session, the patient persistently asks to schedule her analytic hours, as a vital need in her psychic world to find concrete support in the analyst's response. Jasmine's several silent motor reactions are felt by the analyst as feelings of sadness. Moreover, 'the feelings of futility and the grey' in the patient's life illustrate some traits of the clinical picture of melancholy.

In contrast to the analyst's intense countertransference feelings, the patient continues talking about 'fun and good times with work' in order to defensively conceal her true feelings. I think that Marina Perris's observation that the outburst of rage and desire 'to undo her life in a fury', and her related fear of losing 'all that matters', are closely connected to the presence of an early traumatic 'loss' of the maternal function. In the beginning of the analysis, the acute, lethal, abdominal pain seems to be a repetition of the symptom of 'tummy aches' that the patient had experienced during her primary school years. This somatic symptom may indicate the reactivation of a traumatic situation that stems from the analyst's lack of physical affection because of the limitations of the analytic setting. The absence of physical affection elicits feelings of worry and uncertainty about the analyst's desire for her, as did her mother's absence during her childhood. From her memories of the maternal family of origin, we can keep in mind her repetitive feeling of not being welcome, of being excluded from the family. The repetitive daydream of her death after being hit by a car near her home, and the image of her mother crying and screaming, express the fantasy of a very violent, sadomasochistic relationship with the mother.

Theoretical discussion

I think that McDougall's position on patients suffering from breast cancer is very interesting. The author argues that the loss of the breast means that the essential symbol of femininity is felt to be destroyed. On a psychic level, the consequences could be feelings of loss of bodily integrity, disturbances in self-image and a sense of subjective identity, as well as perturbation in the feeling of sexual identity. Therefore, apart from the obvious threat of death, there are additional feelings of confusion in relation to others, as well as anxious feelings concerning sexual and love relations. With regard to the analytical treatment, McDougall stresses: 'An important aspect of psychoanalytic work with breast cancer patients is the revelation of the nature of their ties to their own mothers, which is frequently found to be a highly disturbed relationship' (McDougall, 2004, p. 10).

It is undeniably a matter of clinical observation that in certain cases a significant object loss is associated after a period of time with the development of a somatic illness. It seems that in these cases the loss disrupts the pre-existing unstable psychosomatic equilibrium and homeostasis. Marty and the Paris Psychosomatic School suggest that there is a strong connection between a traumatogenic loss event and the subject's psychosomatic disorganisation. Therefore, trauma is defined by the final disorganising effect that it brings about both on psychic and bodily integrity. According to this psychosomatic approach, the failure of the psyche's capacities for adaptation reveals the present activity of traumatism.

In the same line of thought, Claude Smadja, in his interesting study under the title 'Deuil, mélancholie et somatisation' (Smadja, 2013), explores some specific characteristics of somatisation. By comparing three clinical reactions to the loss of a real or imaginary object, Smadja arrives at the conclusion that somatisation constitutes a somatic solution to the primary narcissistic trauma of a premature ego development. Due to the object loss, the primary narcissistic trauma is reactivated, resulting in psychosomatic essential depression. This is a form of depression which lacks psychic symptoms of the work of mourning as a narcissistic solution, as well as symptoms of the work of melancholy as a masochistic solution. In contrast, in essential depression we frequently observe the appearance of somatic symptoms: psychosomatic disintegration (somatic regression or progressive disorganisation) might be the result of pre-existing non-integration due to multiple splittings. At the same time, at the emotional level there is an absence of feelings of grief. The decathexis of the death drive acts freely and dominates, extinguishing the pain recognition mechanism, which resembles psychic self-mutilation. Due to psychic trauma, the psychic representations, which would allow the binding of the drive, are unavailable and so they are substituted with the presence of the somatic symptoms. Somatic pain substitutes the absent psychic pain, and the ailing body takes charge and stands in for the absent psychic object.

As concerns the internal perception of somatic pain in the organisation of narcissistic cathexes, Freud says: 'Pain seems to play a part in the process and the way in which we gain new knowledge of our organs during painful illnesses and is perhaps a model of the way by which, in general, we arrive at the idea of our body' (1923, pp. 25–26). In this line of thought, we can assume that when a somatic symptom develops, a new somatic object without symbolic meaning develops as well (e.g. Cate's neoplasm and Jasmine's benign cysts); this new somatic object may be sensorially perceived as painful, and the new somatic object may stimulate the psychic apparatus to reinforce narcissistic investments in the body and potentially the psychic work of mentalisation.

It seems that the psychic work of linking the recent object loss with past experiences of loss is defective. The failure of psychic modification as a capacity for adaptation shows up the already present deficiencies at the representational network level. The experience of loss is identified only as a perceptual event without the participation of the whole psychic apparatus, and without the arousal of libidinal and aggressive drives. On the contrary, it seems that the disobjectalising function of the death drive, which according to Green is a radical form of negativity (Green, 2005, p. 121), is dominant.

More specifically, in the case of somatisation it seems that the loss of the external object causes significant modifications to biological functions. It is as if the sensory perception of change in external reality provokes changes in the reality of bodily functions without the participation of the dynamic and creative functioning of the drives. This coincides in a way with Marty's emblematic statement: 'The unconscious receives but does not send' (Marty, 1980, p. 63). The mechanism of splitting within the ego keeps the traumatic cores active, like fragility zones inside the psychosomatic unity.

Moreover, with regard to the loss and its effects on a bodily level, the question that arises is the importance that the lost object had for the subject before its loss, i.e. the role of the object's presence in the subject's psychosomatic equilibrium, since its loss causes the subject's disorganisation. I think that this issue can be illuminated by Freud: 'For the Ego perception plays the part which in the Id falls to instinct. The Ego represents what may be called reason and common sense, in contrast to the Id which contains the passions' (Freud, 1923, p. 25).

Obviously, Freud refers to the conscious part of the ego, since he includes perception, reason and common sense; he juxtaposes this with the unconscious part of the Ego, which originates in and remains related to the reservoir of drives, the Id – where passions take place.

By rendering perception as valuable as the drives, Freud upgrades perception to an energy supplier to the ego, and through the ego to the psychic whole. Clinical observations about the particular value that perception has for so-called psychosomatic patients seem to converge in seeing it as an energy supplier to the ego cut off from its unconscious roots. In a similar way, using the Winnicottian theory of breakdown, Press refers to 'a drive life which was imperfectly embodied, which has been *cut off from its roots'* (Press, 2013, my italics). Perhaps the hypercathexis of the sensory organs to the perception of the external object serves as a substitute for the deficient presence of the drive objects in the psychic world. The presence of the stimulating perceptible object constitutes the vital support for the subject due to the impoverishment of his/her representational life. Cate's emotional cathexis to her breast cancer urged her to ask for help. In the same way, Jasmine's hypercathexis to her benign cysts resulted in the intensification of the transference-countertransference relationship. In this way, as long as the perceptible object is present, there is supply to the ego preserving the temporarily psychosomatic balance and preventing the breakdown. But when the perceptible object disappears, the supply to the ego disappears as well, and so there emerges the early deficiency in the representational-symbolic chain within the ego. The traumatic lack of an internalisation, and symbolisation process, which should have taken place while the object was still alive and before its total and definitive loss, is emphasised.

JÖRG FROMMER

The relationship between trauma and psychosomatics is twofold. On the one hand, traumatic events – especially those which happen in early childhood – always play an important role in the pathogenesis of psychosomatic disorders. On the other hand, serious somatic symptoms irrespective of their origin are always a threatening experience and can thus often be perceived as traumatic in themselves. Consequently, like many other psychosomatic cases, the cases of Jasmine and Cate show an overwhelming *too much* of excitation in terms of fear, free-floating anxiety, and other negative affects, especially in the initial situation. At the same time, these patients displayed a significant *not enough* of symbolisation in terms of being able to find thoughts, metaphors, and phrases to describe their inner lives in interpersonal communications.

I would not go so far as to claim that this paradoxical combination of *over-excitation* and *under-symbolisation* is specific to psychosomatic patients. In some psychosomatic patients, the excitation is masked, and the patient does not seem to appear very excited over long periods of treatment. For instance, only physiological tests like blood pressure might indicate what is going on behind the scenes. And certainly, in many patients without somatic symptoms caused by physiological dysfunctions or structural organ damage, excitation also plays a central role. So, regarding the question of specificity, I would suggest that psychosomatic patients do not present completely different psychic structures to non-psychosomatic patients. Rather, I would say that they present a *too much of excitement* in combination with a *not enough of symbolisation*, and they do so more prominently than other patients; thus, psychosomatic patients are more suitable for the study of these paradoxical states.

What are the roots of suffering from an excess of excitement that is not able to be contained by the symbolisation capacity? To answer this question, I would like to stress the similarities between psychosomatic patients and trauma patients. Both kinds of patients experience a flooding of negative emotions, and the beginning of the treatment is often characterised by a re-enactment of this flooding. The flooding has deep roots in the patient's life history, but it is also caused and reactivated by actual life events. In psychosomatic and trauma patients, the over-excitation occurs in a more specific manner than in neurotic cases, and it becomes manifest not only in different forms of anxiety, but also in fear.

Anxiety and fear as causes of over-excitation in psychosomatic patients

In my view, the *anxiety aspect* represents the reactivation of the early non-availability of a good-enough mother relationship. The mother's failure to aid the child's affect regulation in early infancy leads to a defective capacity for affect perception, affect differentiation, and affect expression. As a result, what the Paris School describes as *operative thinking* arises (Aisenstein and Rappoport de Aisemberg, 2010). From a Winnicottian perspective, the frustration of the need to be held by a secure and loving maternal caretaker in situations of negative excitement and desperation, leads to the destruction of the transitional object which cannot survive. This traumatisation results in the persistence of an omnipotent self that does not allow independent objects to exist (Oliner, 2015; Winnicott, 1971). The flipside of keeping the whole world under the control of your omnipotent self is an empty world without independent objects that can help overcome loneliness. From my perspective, it makes sense to integrate different concepts within psychoanalysis, including empirical research, in order to describe these deficits in mentalisation.

Whereas anxiety plays a central role in neurosis too, in psychosomatic and trauma patients fear is an additional burden. In my view, anxiety is mainly triggered by pre-oedipal and oedipal intra-psychic causes, whereas fear is caused by 'extra-psychic' dangers, i.e. dangers from the actual physical and social world. The difference between anxiety and fear is that fear is adequate to the actual life situation – most other people would feel the same way in the same life situation – whereas with anxiety, dangers perceived to be in the external world are mainly caused by defences against libidinal and aggressive affects. This leads us to the difficulties that some analysts have with the concepts of physical, biological and social *reality*. While it wasn't the case for Freud, for some colleagues nowadays the internal psychic world of the patient and the intra-psychic world of the analyst's countertransference are the dominant players in psychoanalysis, and the patient's conviction that reality is important is often only seen as a defence against insights into their unconscious conflicts.

Thus, working with somatically ill and/or traumatised patients often challenges the self-understanding of the analyst. If the analyst acknowledges the importance of a real threat to the patient's life, the analyst could achieve a new understanding of the importance of being a helpful object in assisting the patient with affect regulation. The analyst would then better understand why a patient was in need of intra-psychic defence mechanisms, such as massive denials of aspects of reality, in order to stabilise a narcissistic balance. In such cases, psychoanalysis would do better to refrain from the classical interpretation of ego-defence mechanisms. This does not mean that the trauma caused by a severe somatic illness would not lead to neurotic coping mechanisms that are amenable to classical analysis. Often the analyst has to be sensitive to both types of phenomena: the overexcited desperation and deep loneliness which indicate the absence of a holding maternal object, and the neurotic symptoms which show the need for interpretations of defence.

Discussion of the cases

In my discussion of the two cases, I would like to focus on two aspects which seem to me essential to the treatment of psychosomatic patients: first, the handling of traumatic free-floating fear and anxiety; second, the handling of resistance (especially denial and repression) in the transference-countertransference relationship. Both aspects, which are closely interconnected, should be understood as epiphenomena of impairment in the capacity for symbolisation. The treatment techniques proposed for these patients anticipates the danger of traumatic flooding by real fear (caused by somatic symptoms), and/or by neurotic anxiety, and accepts the therapist's responsibility for regulation of the patient's negative affects.

Jasmine

The patient is described as an intelligent, attractive woman in her mid-forties, a successful lawyer who at the beginning of the analysis appears as rushed, in a hurry. She developed her narcissistic equilibrium mainly through identification with her father with whom she felt a special closeness that 'she had enjoyed all her life', thereby compensating for the lack of a positive introjection of her mother, which resulted in vulnerability in the female parts of herself. Later in her life, especially in her professional career as a lawyer, she learned to perfectly hide this vulnerability behind the mask of a tough person who could stand on her own feet.

During the analysis, a sense of precariousness and fragility emerged, resulting from the early experience of being a baby to a mother who was not expecting to have another child. After six years of analysis, characterised by positive transference and idealisation of the analyst, the patient developed somatic symptoms in terms of stress, tinnitus, vertigo, exhaustion, pervasive anxiety, hypertension, tachycardia and recurrent benign cysts in her breast. Interpreting these symptoms somatically, one could assume that the patient's process of identification with the female analyst, which helped her to develop positive female parts of herself, was complicated by the patient's own ageing process, characterised by a loss of female attractiveness. Thus, we see the paradoxical coincidence of Jasmine's emerging positive cathexis of the female aspects of her body and self, and the emergence of the psychic and somatic vulnerability of this part of her identity.

The sessions with Jasmine are full of anxiety due to the real risk that the breast cyst might be diagnosed as cancer. To make an appointment for a second opinion of the cyst, the patient cancels her Friday session with the analyst. In the session that follows the missed session, the patient complains about 'just more waiting' without specifically explaining what she means. The analyst's interpretation that follows connects this 'waiting' not with the breast examination, but with what she describes as the 'longer waiting than usual for your session today'. Thus, the analyst picks up on the patient's wish for a close relationship with the analyst as a central theme, expressed by the patient's fantasy of 'grabbing your arm'. This interpretation is useful for the analysis of the neurotic roots of the patient's anxiety as a defence against an eroticised need for physical closeness in the transference, and her wish that the analyst will respond to her person, and especially to the female parts of her body, which is accompanied by massive shame affects. In the third session, this fruitful analytic process enables the patient's dream, which unveils the incident with her cousin when she was around eleven years old. All in all, the cancer anxiety is analysed as part of a defence against neurotic *libidinal anxiety* (Freud, 1923, p. 58), caused by a split off, traumatic, early sexual experience.

Cate

The second patient seems to be similar to Jasmine in many regards. She is in her mid-forties too, self-sufficient; she grew up with a non-empathic mother, has a close relationship with her father, and the meetings with the analyst begin with a much excitation. But despite these similarities, a main contrast resonates from the first moment. Cate's problem is not cancer anxiety boosted by hypochondriac feelings, but the fear or *realistic anxiety* (Freud, 1923, p. 58), of dying of the cancer that has already been diagnosed in her breast, which involves three lymph gland metastases. The fear of this threat is overwhelming and the analyst's feeling, right from the first telephone conversation, that there is something atypical about this case, could have caused the Freudian slip over not hearing the doorbell.

Metapsychological and clinical reflections

According to Freud's second theory of anxiety, metapsychologically one could say that *furcht* or 'fear' in my terminology, which is identical to *realangst* (translated as 'realistic anxiety' by Joan Riviere; Freud, 1923, p. 58) indicates that the patient's ego gives up the libidinal cathexis of the body because this body is sick with cancer (it is a 'bad' body). Due to the close relationship between the ego and the body, this loss of libidinal cathexis of the body means that 'the ego gives itself up because it feels hated and persecuted by the super-ego, instead of loved' (Freud, 1923, p. 58), resulting in what Freud calls *todesangst* (translated as 'fear of death'; Freud, 1923, p. 58).

In this situation, Cate's analyst reacts completely differently to Jasmine's analyst. He acknowledges that the ego-defence has broken down and that the patient has regressed under the pressure of anxiety and fear to the level of primitive presymbolic interaction. This deep form of regression threatens the analyst too, and it forces him to unconsciously protect his competence as a reliable, mature, and separate ego by suppressing his feelings of danger and disorganisation. What results as a conscious feeling is the 'fantasy of non-existent help in our relationship', according to Fotis Bobos. In this situation, the very concrete physical enactment of giving the patient a handkerchief to dry her tears could be understood as a *joining*, which ensures the patient that: *(a) there is somebody, (b) this person does something helpful, (c) this happens on a level of psychic functioning, which fits the actual level of the patient's mentalisation capacity*. Thus, the analyst enables the patient to re-establish the libidinal cathexis of their body, and he offers support to the ego to survive the threat of fear of death caused by the realistic anxiety of losing the object – 'my own body'.

Whereas the analysis of Jasmine reveals the neurotic conflict behind the cancer phobia through the interpretation of repressed libidinal wishes, the analyst of Cate offers a 'cosy nest' for the traumatised patient, which allows her to gradually integrate the destructive and self-destructive fantasies and feelings, which were not only caused by the illness, but as Fotis argues, may have had an influence in the formation of the cancer.

Commentary

BÉRENGÈRE DE SENARCLENS

Both authors insist on the role of primary trauma in the pathogenesis of psychosomatic disorder. Trauma is defined as a 'too much' of excitement and a 'not enough' of symbolisation, something which exceeds the ego's capacities. Fotis adds that trauma represents the disorganising effect on the psychic and somatic apparatus. Jörg argues that somatic patients present this 'too much – not enough' in a more paradoxical combination than other patients. Both state how actual life events can reactivate archaic traumas and how bodily symptoms could be an expression of this. They link trauma with a failure in the primary encounter or with what Bion would call a deficient alpha function in the mother. It seems that, in this case, the kind of *folie à deux* featured in the early days of the mother–baby relationship somewhat fails and is then endlessly searched for.

Jörg insists on the splitting process, illustrating how negative emotions generated by early traumas can be contained in a split and thereby maintained as active as alive. Since it can be reactivated, this split represents a zone of fragility in the psychosomatic balance. It points towards a defence against an overwhelming form of anxiety. Jörg differentiates between anxiety pertaining to neurotic patients and nameless dread which applies to somatising patients. This dread seemingly relates to an unrepresentable fear of death, embedded in the split.

Jörg insists that traumatic experience can be caused by the unexpected somatic symptoms. This raises the question: in such cases, would somatisation be the cause of trauma or its consequence? For Fotis, the patient's reaction to an actual illness is greatly influenced by early trauma and the way it was dealt with. But Jörg's position seems hesitant on this point: giving the example of cancer or multiple sclerosis, he insists on the fact that fear can be caused by extra-psychic dangers, dangers in the real physical and social world. However, he later agrees that the fear of an illness is related to the entire construction of the individual, to their prior responses to traumatic events, and to their introjection – or not – of a sufficiently reliable object.

It is undeniable that for too long psychoanalysis has not paid enough attention to social, physical and biological reality. We know how essential it is to consider both internal and external reality within a kind of equilibrium. Interestingly, when confronted with the clinical material, both authors seem convinced that if the patient cannot feel that both their psychic and external realities are acknowledged in the treatment, the analytic process becomes thwarted, somehow repeating the primary trauma.

Both authors mention the importance of perception for psychosomatic patients. Fotis is more specific. For him, perception can be an energy supplier for an ego cut-off from its drive roots. He adds that the hypercathexis of the sensory and perceptive aspects of the external object serves as a substitute for the deficient presence of the drive object in the inner world. The internal object is not integrated as permanent, so the patient clings instead to perception. Early traumas break links, and in this splitting process objects are lost; in this way, the organisation of the symbolisation process gets interrupted. No creation inside the self can stand for something deficient and invisible outside. Jörg also stresses that the loss of the sensory and perceptive aspects of the external object causes significant modifications to biological functions, which can result in somatisations.

Fotis mentions that somatic pain is a substitute for the absence of psychic pain, grief, or mourning emotions. Somatisation comes instead of a psychic breakdown, as a kind of physical 'depression'. Jörg specifies that under drive-related pressure, the third or the transitional object disappears and cannot play its part. The patient regresses to a one-to-one relationship, or to the oneness of the omnipotent ideal ego of the past. This reminds me of Green's suggestion that doing analysis is like learning how to count to three; the patient goes back to one because of regression. It seems that trauma somehow consists of the loss of an innate feeling of continuity and of an internal object. Is that what is persecutory? Somatisation might consequently arise when discontinuity occurs. This suggests to me a clear link between traumatic loss and illness. Some patients express a kind of 'I am sick, so I am alive', which implies that illness could be a strange way of getting in touch with drive-related excitement. Referring to Smadja, Fotis agrees that somatisation constitutes a kind of solution resulting from the primary narcissistic trauma in a premature ego. Green adds that an unremitting ideal ego is internalised in that premature ego. This certainly impairs the quality and strength of the ego.

Discussing Marina's case, Fotis states that bodily symptoms appear as an opening gesture in the analysis. He felt that these early somatisations are a kind of warning about what is contained in the split. Both authors of this chapter agree that somatisation had a useful function in the two cases presented; it somehow *permitted* a call for help. They point to the key importance of the countertransference when dealing with such patients. With hope and despair, it seems that the patients come to analysis and show something that they have no knowledge of. Clearly, the dissonance of their psychic organisation is felt in the countertransference. It somehow plays the role of a third term. The patients' unconscious traumas are often unfurled and inferred from some kind of bodily countertransference in the analyst.

Jörg proposes two axes in working with such patients. The first one consists in attending to the neurotic conflict, through the interpretation of the repressed libidinal wishes and traumatic anxiety. The second one is a handling of the resistance by offering a 'cosy nest' to allow the traumatised patient to integrate destructive fantasies. He speaks of regulating the negative affects through adequate interventions. Is this a matter of proposing representations or constructions? Is this a way of speaking about the necessity of trying to unfold a concealed negative transference, which could be poisonous if left untouched? Jörg affirms that an act by the analyst (such as the offering of a handkerchief) can foster symbolisation and re-establish a libidinal cathexis of the body.

These comments made me think of the great heterogeneity in the structure of somatic patients. Could this be their specificity? Their oedipal organisation is unstable and, as Fotis adds, the psychic elaboration of the conflictual relation with the mother is obstructed. In this respect, it is as if we have to listen to them with two eyes, at their various levels of functioning, in perpetual motion. We have to adapt to this heterogeneity.

Note

1 Marty suggests that certain character neuroses are susceptible to destabilising the economical equilibrium creating a progressive disorganisation (1980, p. 11).

References

Aisenstein, M. and Rappoport de Aisemberg, E. (2010) *Psychosomatics Today: A Psychoanalytic Perspective*. London: Karnac.

Ferenczi, S. (1932) *Final Contributions to the Problems and Methods of Psychoanalysis*. London: Karnac, 1994.

Freud, S. (1892) 'Sketches for the "Preliminary communication" of 1893', in *S.E., Vol. 1*. London: The Hogarth Press, pp. 145–54.

Freud, S. (1914) 'On narcissism: an introduction', *S.E., Vol. 14*. London: The Hogarth Press, pp. 67–102.

Freud, S. (1923) *The Ego and the Id*, in *S.E., Vol. 19*. London: The Hogarth Press, pp. 1–66.

Freud, S. (1939) *Moses and Monotheism: Three Essays*, in *S.E., Vol. 23*. London: The Hogarth Press, pp. 1–138.

Green, A. (2005) *Key Ideas for a Contemporary Psychoanalysis. Misrecognition and Recognition of the Unconscious*. New York: Routledge.

Marty, P. (1980) *L'ordre psychosomatique*. Paris: Payot, pp. 9–124; pp. 137–57.

McDougall, J. (2004) 'The Psychoanalytic Voyage of a Breast-Cancer Patient', *The Annual of Psychoanalysis*, 32, pp. 9–28.

Oliner, M. (2015) 'Weitere untersuchungen über Winnicotts konzept der "objektverwendung"', *Psyche*, 69, pp. 1033–45.

Press, J. (2013) 'Some lines of research', *Communication to Members of the Working Party*.

Smajda, C. (2001) *La vie opératoire. Études psychanalytiques*. Paris: Presses Universitaires de France, pp. 36–43.

Smadja, C. (2013) 'Deuil, mélancholie et somatisation', *Revue française de psychosomatique*, 44, pp. 7–24.

Winnicott, D.W. (1971) *Playing and Reality*. New York: Basic Books.

Chapter 3

Somatic and borderline states

BÉRENGÈRE DE SENARCLENS

There is obviously an intimate connection, a unity, between body and mind. Although they are functionally separate, they work in tandem. However, psychoanalysts first favoured neurotic patients for analysis. A specific interest in borderline psychology, as well as in patients with somatic symptoms, developed only later. But for quite some time it was considered inappropriate to offer a formal treatment to patients with somatic symptoms; the same went for borderline patients, essentially because of their tendency to act out. This trend was slowly reversed, and the fact that these patients were offered the couch led to a change in perspective on technique. It also led to new theoretical reflections, which in turn influenced the clinical work. The clinical work was described as being 'on the edge of analysability'. It underlined the importance of the work of the countertransference and of the sensory material emerging throughout the treatment but primarily in the very first sessions.

Nevertheless, it seems to me that today we cannot speak of a specific way of working with these categories of patients. Our identity as analysts is the only 'compass' to guide us when approaching such pathologies, to help us tolerate their chaos and grasp the unexpected and unrepresented material that emerges. Granted, somatisation processes concern us all. Moreover, we all have to die and our bodies are doomed to become sick and deteriorate throughout life. However, the question remains: why is it that some patients somatise easily and others, rather, have a tendency to act out? This is the point raised in this chapter.

By the term 'borderline states', I mean patients whose structure is heterogeneous, fluctuating. The construction of their identity has been problematic and left them with porous and labile borders, which often makes relationships problematic. As I write these lines, I have in mind the clinical cases presented in this book. Both seem to belong to the category of patients that André Green called 'borderline states' (*états limites*). However, Jasmine seems more depressive but more organised psychically than Cate, who presents a particular tendency to act out. We see that they both somatise, but they have different types of symptomatology:

a more functional one in Jasmine's case, and a more severe pathology as demonstrated by Fotis's case.

At this stage I will try to point out some similarities between borderline or somatising patients, and then some differences. Both patients seem to communicate in peculiar and puzzling ways, beyond words, showing difficulty symbolising. It is as if they were suddenly deprived of more secondary tools. In the cases presented, and in others, can we 'hear' physical symptoms or 'acting-out' as ways of trying to symbolise? Can we envisage both as indicative of very primitive material seeking to be endowed with meaning? As we know, this proposition has often been put into question.

However, in such patients, it seems as if traces of the past had been felt and preserved, but not psychically integrated. The subject is trying to escape through any means the extreme pain that is hidden in them. But it appears that these poorly organised sensations and perceptions – which paradoxically seem as unforgettable as they are impossible to remember – are *knocking on the door* in search of visibility and integration at last. Sometimes it looks as if the compulsion to repeat contains some kind of unconscious intentionality and acts like a 'tool' to elaborate and master what had overwhelmed the capacities of the primitive ego. Along the same lines, Ogden suggests that the *force* which pushes patients to find the source of their anxieties lies in the feeling that they were deprived of essential and vital aspects of their personality due to an early split (Ogden, 2007). Analysts have to 'hear' these strange languages and do something with them.

Could some of the acting-out 'symbolise' an early break or an unbearable pressure? Would a fragile body reflect the failure of a primary encounter? Both could be attempts at representing a 'too much' that was not metabolised in a primitive ego, since it had no adequate psychic defence. We could also raise the question of whether somatisation in the course of analytic treatment could be seen as a bodily figuration of an emotion. In that respect, it could be a very significant movement in the analysis. I wondered about that in the case of Jasmine.

We should of course be careful to avoid generalisations. Somatisations are plural and diverse, and undoubtedly our hypotheses cannot be fully validated in empirical terms. However, apart from their difficulty in symbolising, it seems that these two categories of patients often show a poorly unified ego, narcissistic and identity problems, as well as, occasionally, traces of primary depression. Their destructiveness seems linked to a constraining 'ideal ego'. We could imagine that the violent drive-related tension that suddenly arises could be tied to a disturbing gap between a strong narcissistic ideal ego and reality; the cases of Cate and Jasmine illustrate this.

Sometimes these difficulties are not so visible, and the subject is quite adjusted, but the system breaks down under sensitive circumstances. This seems to be the case with Jasmine. Ferenczi already stressed that as soon as the 'psychic system fails, the organism begins to think' (Ferenczi, 1932, p. 6), or generate enactments. One could wonder whether a fragile and fragmented ego would favour one of these two paths, somatic or behaviour – whereas a well-structured and stable ego would not lead to these developments.

As already stated, trauma is a central issue in these pathologies. It is what overwhelms the psychic capacity of the subject. Trauma reveals the importance of the 'economic' factor. And if there is no object to receive and contain this excess of excitement, there will be no transformation into intelligibility and no accession to any system of representation. Ejection is necessary, and it could favour propulsion into the body or 'acting-out'. Considering mentalisation as the mind's ability to do the work of interpreting, we could argue that the dismantling of mental functioning under the effect of traumatic factors could give rise to acting-out or somatic symptoms.

Let us now try to grasp some differences between these pathologies. I think one difference might be related to activity and passivity. While the borderline patient could be seen to be on the line of the active, the patient who somatises might be more in a passive mode, as if there were some kind of submission to an internal persecutor. The borderline patient tends to act out uncontained drive impulses, whereas the somatic patient tends to suppress all expression of drive or conflict. In this respect, it seems that 'essential depression' would be correlated with that suppression.

In any case, it seems clear that the way of dealing with drives is different. With both types of patients, there is some kind of 'short cut' of the drive: in one case, the drive tension loses itself into the body (the violence being acted in the body), and in the other case, it is expelled via certain forms of behaviour (acting-out). It seems that these are the different prices to be paid for the excitement to abate, as if it could not be elaborated in a more secondary way. Concerning somatisation, we could wonder whether this *losing* into the body could be envisioned as a way of avoiding the object, and maybe the patient's own subjectivity as well. In other words, the somatic symptom could be some kind of a *solution* to avoid the psychic acknowledgement of a non-symbolised but unforgettable trauma?

I would now like to venture the hypothesis of another difference between these patients. For this purpose, I need to make a detour and go back to the construction of the ego in more detail. We observe that the sensations of the baby arise from various sources: visual, auditory, olfactory, tactile and other; these should all be compatible so as to form the first sense of unity, the root feeling of 'being'. But some obstacles can compromise this very first identity or ego unity. At the beginning for the infant there is no sense of self, no difference between outside and inside. The process of the child's psychic transformation starts in the bodily relationship with the mother. Her 'capacity for dreaming' will open and stimulate, contain and signify, the emotional experiences of the newborn child. This work implies an encounter between two psyches, a mutual transformation. Little by little, this encounter will allow the child to fully feel that he exists in a continuum. Sometimes it takes a long time until he is convinced that the object exists for him in a continuum too. We know that this feeling of continuity is absolutely necessary to be able to integrate a 'third object', and thus be able to symbolise. If the nucleus of the self develops harmoniously, the drives might be tamed and made knowable through a process of binding by which they become (though always incompletely) representable, allowing for the growth of mental life. This is an essential process since it determines the strength of the subject's organisation. It can lead to a 'well mentalised' ego, and to an adequate ego/non-ego differentiation. But sometimes this is not the case, and the infant's experience of continuity with an object is so unstable that it impairs the construction of their subjectivity. The narcissistic borderline pathologies confront us precisely with a fragility in this construction of their ego. The synthesis of the subject's different parts is weak: some are missing, frozen, split, encrypted, and the patient feels a terrible anxiety when confronted again with what was split off in the first place. When faced with an economic overcharge, the subject regresses to a state of anxiety in which the borders between subject and object are no longer clear. There are neither two, nor three: sometimes all there is an undifferentiated oneness.

We know that the 'construction' of the ego is linked to the infantile drive activity, as well as to the reaction of the environment. This brings us to Winnicott and his notion of a good enough mother, neither too present, nor too absent. Here again, if this balance is inadequate, the constitution of a structured and differentiated self can be jeopardised. This pertains to both borderline states and somatising patients. To try to differentiate them, I want to stress how the strength of the ego would be the result of a good enough 'work of anality' insofar as the elaboration of the anal stage is key in the evolution and coherence of the ego. The anal stage is a pivotal period of strong stimulations, during which the relation with others and with oneself changes. It is also a time of possible healing, in the 'après-coup' of the oral stage experiences that precede it. It is a time when the child has to make up a narcissistic base. But sometimes this does not happen and instead the child constructs disabling defences, which leave him with feelings of discontinuity, void and violence.

In 1950, Robert Fliess (Fliess, 1950), the son of W. Fliess, used the term 'divided line' to refer to a sort of 'tipping point' between neurotic and non-neurotic structures. He located it at the time of what he called the anal organisation; it is a *divided line* between pregenital and genital structuration and is central to the forthcoming oedipal development. Borderline patients seem to navigate between the two sides of this line, as if their neurotic structuration were not stable. J. Bergeret (Bergeret, 1995) describes them as having a kind of ambiguous, inhibiting fixation on that line, as if they were balancing between psychotic and neurotic organisations.

In his article 'Primary Anality' (Green, 1993), Green also shows the links between borderline patients and some 'avatars' of anality, and he claims that the nature of their investments is primarily narcissistic. He speaks of 'oranality' to show how emotional avidity and traces of the oral relation still infiltrate anality. The child's wound is not healed, and it provokes great pain and constant excitement. He links it to a fear of intrusion and abandonment.

But what does all this mean specifically for somatic patients? Recently, Roussillon proposed the hypothesis of a 'melancholic core' in psychosomatic ailments (Roussillon, 2016, pp. 62–63), which he linked to oral incorporation processes, to something in orality that the later anal experiences could not change or 'repair' (Roussillon, 2016). He thinks that:

> . . . this precipitated in the subject the constitution of a zone of bodily fragility, bearing the scar of some unintegrated subjective experiences. So the body 'speaks'; and it speaks from where the shadow of the object fell on the body. It speaks from a zone of bad primary differentiation. But it speaks 'in the body', in the language of the body. It tells the story of primary disillusions . . . and of the absence of mirroring by the primary object.
>
> (Roussillon, 2016, p. 62)

In Roussillon's view, somatisation would contain an 'hallucinatory activation' of traces of a very early 'bodily' trauma (idem). I think the point raised by Roussillon is a very important one when we try to differentiate between somatic and borderline patients. A failure in this rather primitive oral development of the subject might foster some somatic fragility. The pain might have fixed something in the soma which could not be transformed into thought. It seems that this would be the result of irreparable trauma, which is then severely ejected.

Could we conclude that some categories of somatic ailments are often related to something very early dating back to oral times, something that could not be elaborated or integrated, could not develop harmoniously, and which, finally, gets propelled into the body? Conversely, borderline patients that do not somatise might have failed and frustrating experiences dating back to a later developmental period, pertaining mainly to anal issues. It is true that, quite often, these patients adapt normally to life. But it seems that they keep a very sensitive early wound or early split, which under stressful and emotional circumstances could 'wake up' again forcefully. As we saw, some non-mentalised zones seem to pave the way for somatisation or acting-out, depending on where the fragility zone originates.

CHRISTIAN SEULIN

Somatic pathologies are the inevitable future of all mankind, as innate biological programmes set the temporal limits of human functioning. However, some patients develop acute somatic disorders – in either critical or chronic form – which can be linked to distinct modalities of psychic functioning. I would like to tackle the question of the common features in psychic functioning between the somatising patients and borderline patients. From the outset, there appear to be three clinical characteristics in common: the place of the traumatism in the patients' history, the disorders pertaining to associativity, and the deficiencies in symbolisation during the sessions. Experience also teaches us that somatic disorders frequently arise in borderline patients in periods of crisis. Such crises reflect the sudden advent of some energetic imbalance as a result of the failure of the regular modalities of defence via behaviour, relational drama, or satisfactions of a perverse type.

Both in the case of somatising patients and borderline patients, the psychic elaboration of the drive-related pressure is deficient or obstructed, which means that the action of the drive will take on the basic form of excitation in the soma or in behaviour, circumventing the psychic unfurling of the drive. This might be the most remarkable parallel between somatising patients and borderline patients. The economic viewpoint highlights an energetic overload whose main source is equivocal. In borderline patients, the 'chaotic manifestations of the transference' (Green, 2002, p. 66) frequently reveal how much these patients struggle to develop the drive-object link within a continuity able to generate representative life with its ramified narrative figures.

The inefficiency of the oedipus complex, of the castration complex, and of primal fantasies accounts for the failure of repression, as well as the pathology of the limits (*la double limite*; Green, 1982) between the id and the ego and between the ego and the external world. But what is deficient in the borderline patient is the underlying operation of double reversal (reversal on the subject himself, and between activity and passivity), which is tied to an inability to organise the primal scene fantasy. In these clinical situations, active, passive and excluded third term positions are not symbolised. Such structural inefficiency leads the subject destitute when faced with the pressure of the drive, which lacks any framework to express itself, that is to say, to attenuate the pressure through the work of binding. It is consequently subject to a sudden discharge, which operates as a short-circuit into the registers of emotion and behaviour.

We recognise here characteristics featured in the case of Cate whose impulsive behaviour, alcohol addiction, and erratic sexual relationships, long served as a path for drive-related gratification. It seems that the loss of external landmarks and forms of support – a fulfilling job, a young and still dependent son, physical attractiveness – might have meant the loss of possibilities of discharge, leading to somatic breakdown.

In many somatising patients, emotional suppression leads the drive to find an outcome in the soma through an extreme process of disqualification of affects that return to a state of senseless excitation, cut off from representational life (Seulin, 2005). If the solution provided by automatic anxiety is not enough, the risk of the drive acting in the soma then manifests itself. Borderline patients are therefore at risk of somatic illness when an energetic overload arises because of a loss or a new traumatism, which cannot be curbed through recourse to behavioural and relational crises, impulses, or addictions.

In patients at risk of major somatisation, the same phenomenon of energetic overload is at play, caused in such cases by the suppression of the drives and a lack of drive-related qualification, or by the breakdown of splitting, so that the ego becomes overwhelmed. There is no release in relational life or in the external world, and the quantum acts on the soma. In Jasmine's case, it seems that the breakdown of a form of ego splitting caused the ego to become invaded by large quantities of unqualified, nameless energy, and this played a part in the emergence of the organic disorders (breast cysts).

The two categories of patients can also be considered from the perspective of object relations. For both patients, the object is not recognised as another subject whose distinct desires and actions lead to a disappointment when they fail to coincide with the patient's primarily narcissistic expectation. The dynamics of idealisation and depreciation reflects the narcissistic utilitarian demand that the patient imposes upon the object. We are aware that in allergic structures and in illnesses involving flare-ups, separation can be experienced as wrenching (Marty, 1958). What is referred to as 'essential depression' at the root of somatic disorganisations, considered to be a form of objectless depression, seems to stem rather from an irreparable disappointment caused by the object, which leads to a negative narcissistic withdrawal. The borderline patient can be recognised in this scenario, even though, unable to endure the object loss, he or she long strove to sustain an objectal link involving drama or instability, wavering between disappointment and idealisation.

In the countertransference, the assessment of operative thinking appears as a form of objectification which I call 'a transference of no transference': the complete loss of hope in an object causes the patient to refuse to invest in an object, and the object is experienced with the certainty of not expecting anything. This type of transference comes with the necessary repetition of a compulsive and recurring form of attachment to the negative dimension of the primary object. In this case, as with the melancholic subject, the known, negative, and deadly dimension of the object – as the subject's eradicator – counts because of its permanence. It is not the quality of the link that matters, but its permanence and its faithful reproduction of the unconscious parental death wish.

I am in general agreement with the suggestions that Bérengère de Senarclens makes in her essay. However, I would like to discuss certain points that she makes regarding the differences between borderline patients and somatising patients. First of all, following Jean Bergeret with whom I have had numerous conversations, I think that the borderline patients he describes primarily suffer from separation anxiety. This core of 'depressivity' prevents these patients from depressing fully and from acquiring any stable form of structuring (Bergeret, 1975). They are neither neurotic nor psychotic, but they may develop in either direction, as well as in the area of perversion. Bergeret carefully distinguishes his account of borderline patients from those described by Otto Kernberg (Kernberg, 1975) and Green (Green, 1990) where we are dealing with pre-psychotics at great risk of somatisation. Fliess's 'divided line', which Bergeret often refers to (Bergeret, 1975), separates the primary anal stage from the secondary anal stage, and draws a border between neurosis and psychosis; these differences express, using the theory of stages, the incapacity and capacity for drive introjection and erotic pleasure.

In my view, if we consider the two categories of patients, i.e. borderline patients as pre-psychotic and severely somatising patients, we can say that their capacities for symbolisation are obstructed and the subjective symbolisation of passive and active positions is deficient (Seulin, 2015). Activity and passivity are present, but they both stem from defence measures that are mobilised before the onset of invasion and abandonment anxieties; they merely reflect the biologically innate activity passivity couple, and that the vicissitudes of this innate condition is subjected to environment influences.

Bergeret sees borderline states as raising the issue of fundamental violence (Bergeret, 1984). In this context, the relation to the object is like *the little one facing the big one*, dominated by the implicit murder – implicit for the unconscious – inherent in any form of self-assertion before others. The issue that borderline (described by both Kernberg and Green) and somatising patients both raise is akin to melancholia, in which attachment to the bad object, or to the negative dimension of the object, prevails. Clinging on to the primary object thus carries on indefinitely, as the work of representation of the object never comes to pass, and the inscription of a third always fails. The very origin of the psychic elaboration of the drive is at stake here, which implies living through the attack of the object, an experience only possible when the object has survived and when enough satisfaction has been found in the object relation. Finally, I would like to stress that concerning the main issues, borderline patients and somatising patients seems to me to be very close. Defences may vary, but early traumas, melancholia, threat, and difficulties concerning psychic symbolic elaboration, are at stake in both.

Commentary

MARINA PERRIS-MYTTAS

As noted by Bérengère de Senarclens, the psychoanalytic investigation of borderline pathology started gathering momentum almost concurrently with the start of the development of the psychoanalytic study of patients who somatise. Indeed, from the 1950s onwards we see a vigorous development of psychoanalytic thinking that concerns psychopathology beyond the realm of neurosis. Psychoanalysis is extended, we might say, to the understanding and the treatment of patients whose psychic functioning lies outside the two hypothetical limits of the psychic field: the 'acting' and the 'soma'.

The authors of this chapter explore what they see as the common and diverse features in the psychological make up and history of psychic development of borderline and somatic patients. Furthermore, both authors suggest that we become aware of these features as we get to experience them through our psychoanalytic work with these patients. The authors' agreement about the presence of early trauma in the primary object relation is in my opinion their shared starting point. Trauma is also the hallmark of their shared understanding of these pathologies. So, with trauma as their starting point, both authors emphasise the consequent vicissitudes of the economic aspect of the drive. The economic aspect is pivotal to the authors' understandings of both conditions as well as to their, at times, overlapping clinical pictures.

As a result of the primary traumatism, there is in these patients' psychic functioning an excess of drive movement, which acts as what Christian Seulin refers to as 'a formless excitation': an excitation which is not contained and 'cannot be transformed to intelligibility'. Furthermore, the constitution of the drive gets obstructed and, as Bérengère de Senarclens says, 'there is no accession to a system of representation'. This excess of drive activity overwhelms the capacity for psychic elaboration, and in its place, we see action. This action can take the form of the by now pathognomonic sign of borderline patients: acting-out. Alternatively, the action can be turned inwards and become acting-in in the soma. This leads to the development of somatic symptoms, which we witness in the unfolding of somatic processes when patients fall ill.

Furthermore, both authors agree that the internal situation in which action is the currency of communication results from, as well as further generates, representational gaps, difficulties in psychic elaboration and the work of symbolisation. In this context, Bérengère de Senarclens raises a question which concerns the delimitation of psychic functioning and processing: Could some acting 'symbolise an early rupture or an unbearable pressure?'. That is, can we consider that an act (albeit a form of communication as it might well be) may possibly have the status of a symbol? A symbol either along the trajectory towards the external world, as an *acting-out*, or in the direction of the soma, as an *acting-in* in the soma. This is an interesting question, which in my opinion might open up further inroads into the exploration of both pathologies.

Additional characteristics which are well documented in analytic theory and accounts of clinical work, like a poorly integrated ego, and elements of narcissistic pathology, are recognised by both authors as central to the clinical presentation of borderline and somatic patients. Furthermore, Bérengère de Senarclens emphasises the dominance of a tyrannical ideal ego, heir of primary narcissism, which in these patients partly or totally replaces the oedipal superego with its protective dimensions. Another difference, stressed by this author, is that in borderline patients the fragility of anal organisation is paramount, and not so for somatic patients.

The core common characteristic of both pathologies is understood to concern the object which is not recognised as another subject. With somatic patients, this internal situation can be arrived at, as Bérengère de Senarclens suggests, by the physically ill patients' manner of losing his/her subjectivity into the body. While with borderline patients, Christian Seulin emphasises that the link with the object is maintained through 'drama' and marked by 'an inability to accept object loss'. Against this backdrop, both authors are of the opinion that the principal differences between these two groups of patients lies, par-excellence, in the way that the object relations are formed, shaped and developed. During psychoanalysis the divergence in the nature and the qualities of object relations results in the very different dynamics of the transference and countertransference that these two groups of patients evoke.

More specifically, it is my opinion that the difference in the two pathologies is principally related to the attributes and the nature of the mediating object. The object, that is, who mediates primary experiences and facilitates or hinders the constitution of the drive and the opening up to the world of representations. In my experience, the mediating object which we often encounter in the analysis of borderline states in the patient's narratives, dreams, and through the countertransference, is fragmented and chaotic: the analyst often suffers the object's disturbing fragmentation, especially during periods of stagnation in analysis. In a very different manner, as time goes on the somatic patient's object makes its presence felt in the analyst through the feeling of being intruded upon; with time, we come to experience a multifaceted traumatic intrusiveness, often an infliction of psychic absence, as the object's primary way of relating and communicating through unconscious undercurrents.

In both groups of patients, distance and separation in the primary relationship is experienced as intolerable. Still, the transference formed by these two groups of patients are very dissimilar, almost antithetical we could say, if we are to think of the intensity and contradictory nature of the transference of borderline patients, compared with the apparent absence of alive affectivity and specificity of transference reactions that are characteristic of somatic patients, as described by Marty and the Paris School of Psychosomatics.

References

Bergeret, J. (1984) *La violence fondamentale*. Paris: Dunod.

Bergeret, J. (1975) *La depression et les états-limites*. Paris: Payot.

Bergeret, J. (1995) 'L'analité et la maîtrise', *Revue française de psychanalyse*, 3, pp. 659–82.

Ferenczi, S. (1932) *The Clinical Diary of Sandor Ferenczi*, ed. J. Dupont, trans. M. Balint and N.Z. Jackson. Cambridge, MA: Harvard University Press, 1988.

Fliess, R. (1950) *Symbol, Dream and Psychosis*. New York: International University Press, 1973.

Green, A. (1982) 'La double limite', in Green A. (1990) *La folie privée*. Paris: Gallimard.

Green, A. (1990) *La folie privée*. Paris: Gallimard.

Green, A. (1993) 'L'analité primaire', *Monographies de la revue française de psychanalyse*. Paris: Presses Universitaires de France, pp. 61–86.

Green, A. (2002) *Idées directrices pour une psychanalyse contemporaine*. Paris: Presses Universitaires de France.

Kernberg, O. (1975) *Borderline Conditions and Pathological Narcissism*. Northvale, NJ: Jason Aronson.

Marty, P. (1958) 'La relation objectale allergique', *Revue française de psychanalyse*, 22, 1, pp. 7–30.

Ogden, T.H. (2007) 'On talking-as-dreaming', *Int. J. Psychoanal.*, 88, 3, pp. 575–89.

Roussillon, R. (2016) *Corps parlant, corps parlé, corps muet*. Paris: Editions in Press.

Seulin, C. (2005) 'L'excitation transmise', *Revue française de psychanalyse*, 69, 1, pp. 203–15.

Section III

Treatment

Chapter 4

Psychosomatic investigation and treatment

EVA SCHMID-GLOOR

Even before the 1960s, a number of psychoanalysts had carried out intensive work with patients with psychosomatic illness. Some of those psychoanalysts applied their usual classical technique. However, other clinicians employed a somewhat different technique by introducing new parameters, like taking a supportive or mirroring position. In the end, they were disappointed to find that neither the aetiology nor the pathogenesis of the psychosomatic disorders were really understood and helped by psychoanalytic practice. At the beginning of the 1960s, some of the representatives of the Paris School of Psychosomatics described a 'psychosomatic structure' which they claimed is common to all patients who suffer from psychosomatic illness (Marty, de M'Uzan, and David, 1962). They attributed to these patients 'operatory thinking' and 'operatory life', expressing a 'robotic' kind of mental functioning (Marty, de M'Uzan, and David, 1962), which they viewed as the outcome of a psychic and somatic disorganisation process marked by a state of negativity and undoing of mental functioning.

The German psychoanalyst Johannes Cremerius, among others (for example, Gerd Overbeck), called the Paris School's ideas into question. In the 1970s, Cremerius argued that the theory of the 'psychosomatic structure' (Cremerius, 1977) arose out of the specific investigation interviews that the Paris School undertook. Cremerius pointed out that the patients selected for the Paris School's research project were patients from the Parisian clinics for internal medicine, surgery etc., who did not come to the interview with an explicit wish for analytic treatment. Most of the patients in the interviews exclusively complained of bodily ailments, hoping to be rid of them as soon as possible. Otherwise, they insisted on having no psychological or emotional difficulties whatsoever and no desire for therapy. Cremerius claimed that the 'psychosomatic structure', including symptoms of 'emptiness' and the *pensée operatoire* (operatory thinking) (Marty, de M'Uzan, and David, 1962), could be seen to be specifically linked to interview situations. In his own private practice, Cremerius showed that the psychosomatic patients who voluntarily came to a first interview with the wish for psychoanalytic treatment had not shown the characteristic personality traits as described by the French authors. Cremerius claimed that he worked with psychosomatic patients in the same way as with other patients, and that he could not define specific structural differences between them. I think that Cremerius draws our attention to the fact that even today, questions remain about the kinds of analytic techniques to use with psychosomatic patients.

Marty initially thought that he had found the appropriate technique for psychosomatic patients, claiming that what is most important in the case of an 'operatory' patient is to re-establish the functioning of the preconscious, which he considered to be the central damaged part of the psyche of these patients. In aiming to arrive at an exact diagnostic classification, Marty was running the risk of becoming some kind of 'medical doctor of the psyche', and as a consequence he risked the loss of anchorage in psychoanalysis, and specifically the importance of the countertransference (Press, 2016). Marty might not have paid extensive attention to the countertransference because he developed his theoretical ideas at a time when the concept of the countertransference in France had not yet acquired the same importance as it had in England (Paula Heimann, Donald Winnicott, Wilfred Bion). Nowadays, we could not imagine any psychoanalytical treatment, especially of borderline patients or patients with psychosomatic fragility, without including the countertransference as a crucial tool.

I would now like to bring into focus the issue of the initial interview and the attempt to make a diagnostic evaluation. In our Working Group on Psychosomatics, we have identified interesting and relevant connections between the initial interviews and the later development of the analytic process. Is it possible that through the evaluation of the initial interview we can make hypothetical predictions about the weak points in the psychic structure of the patient that may put them – especially when under pressure – at risk of suffering a future somatic derailment? Addressing such a question means that the analyst must be prepared to be open to the countertransference in the initial interview, which involves the analyst's capacity to address his own areas of anxieties linked to his own bodily-psychosomatic existence and mortality.

In the first interview, Fotis Bobos found his patient's headscarf – a visible 'stigma' of her illness – so disturbing that it provoked in him an immediate rejecting attitude to the patient. It is very likely that on an immediate physical level, this patient provoked in her analyst something akin to a psychic threat, which the analyst could only react to initially with rejection. Considering the analyst's function as a resonating body to the patient's deepest archaic anxieties, could we say that the analyst can be addressed at a preverbal, bodily level?

Marina Perris gives an account of the initial interview with her female patient and her own sense of puzzlement, since she could not understand the patient's wish to undergo analysis. She finally realised that the patient was making every effort to present herself as though she were completely independent and autonomous, because she feared narcissistic injuries from the object. In their first meeting, the patient neither provoked massive anxieties in Marina, nor a rejecting reaction – either on a psychical or bodily level. However, what Marina and her patient will only come to fully realise many years later in the course of the analytic process, is that the patient is only able to get in touch with and integrate deep areas of narcissistic fragility during a phase of massive somatisation.

I would now like to offer a more detailed discussion of the clinical material of Marina's analysis with her female patient. What I think is most remarkable is Marina's capacity to finally mobilise a symbolisation process that helped the patient to get in touch with and formerly integrate non-integrated areas of narcissistic fragility and traumatic vulnerability. When Jasmine suffered from tinnitus, Marina interpreted this as an attempt to fill up her ears with loud noise in order to escape hearing her analyst's voice. Marina interpreted tachycardia as symbolising the first stirrings of amorous love, and she understood the cysts as expressing a deep longing to be touched and looked at tenderly. These interpretations show how Marina creates links that lead to meaningful interpretations by carefully considering her countertransference feelings.

Early on, Marina is able to tolerate the experience of inadequacy and formlessness in the analytic sessions, which she did not prematurely interpret as an identification with the failing internal object. When Jasmine started developing cysts in her breast, which in turn led her to experience dreadful anxiety attacks, deadly terrors, and hypochondria, this phase in the analysis was experienced by the analyst as an impasse or standstill, while at the same Marina understood that the patient had to make the analyst experience a sense of failure, specifically a failure to put an end to the patient's terrible agony. In a brief instance of *reverie* through her countertransference, Marina registered an image of a mother nursing her baby, which to her utter dismay evoked an immediate negative response of disapproval. The analyst was in a position to make use of her countertransference to establish a vital link to the patient's early experiences, when the awakening of her instinctual life and longing for sensual bodily contact were ignored by the object.

Due to the thoughtful and thorough elaboration of the countertransference processes in Marina's analysis of Jasmine, the integration of painful and traumatic aspects of the patient's psychic experience eventually became possible. Can we look into the possibility that this patient's drives would have found a different outlet than somatisation if the patient could have endured the awakening of her drive-life towards her analyst in the transference, instead of in a lateral transference? Or could this traumatised area only be expressed in a *language of the body* because it concerned split-off traumatic experiences, which had taken place in the earliest, pre-verbal period of life. In other words, could this patient only express her early traumatic experiences with the help of this very archaic primary bodily symbolisation? In the course of the analysis, the analytic couple were successful in attributing symbolic meaning to the various somatic symptoms.

It seems that in the case of Marina's patient we can observe – probably due to a re-activation of early narcissistic injuries through the unfolding of the transference – a somatic crisis that had to be endured and survived. Yet in the case of Fotis's patient, a severe and much more threatening somatic breakdown had already occurred when she started treatment, and her psychic conditions seemed very different from those of Marina's patient. In Marina's clinical case, we can see how the analyst's capacity to stay in a passive position is necessary for the creation of a psychic space, which allows the patient – in a certain phase of the analysis – to express her experiences in somatic symptoms; these can then be interpreted, leading to the integration of early traumatic, narcissistic injuries. During the somatic crisis, the experience of the *failing object* is shown to be crucial and has to be experienced by the analytic couple and survived by the analyst. In my view, this kind of analytic process is not specific to a psychosomatic patient but could occur in a rather similar way with a borderline patient.

JACQUES PRESS

The clinical accounts that open the present volume allow us to gauge the work of the Paris Psychosomatic School, as well as touch on the progress that has since been made regarding the process of investigation and the handling of the treatment. As Eva Schmid-Gloor reminds us, between 1960–1980, the founders of the Paris Psychosomatic School developed a specific technique pertaining to initial meetings with somatising patients and their subsequent treatment. The technique is closely linked to a theoretical view of the processes leading to somatic illness. For these authors, somatic illness does not assume any symbolic value, but is instead inscribed in a process of disorganisation that first affects the psyche before progressing to the soma.[1] The first and pivotal step in analysis thus logically consists in examining the factors that might have led to the disorganisation. In this regard, it is highly significant that the founding text of the Paris School should be entitled – and focused on – what they call the 'psychosomatic investigation' (Marty, de M'Uzan and David, 1963). The point of this investigation is to establish with as much accuracy as possible a diagnosis of the 'quality of mental functioning', which in Marty's view is expressed by the quality of preconscious functioning; the investigation then involves highlighting the gaps in this functioning and the way in which traumatic elements might have disorganised it, resulting in somatisation. Once these roots have been established, in the course of the treatment the analyst must implement a stance involving relatively little interpretation. Marty coined the term 'maternal function' to refer to this stance of the analyst (Marty, 1980). In the forthcoming discussion, I will tackle the two stages in question – investigation and treatment – and consider them in relation to Jasmine and Cate.

Psychosomatic investigation

There is a preliminary question that often comes up in discussions – can we anticipate the kinds of somatisation through the Paris School's *psychosomatic investigation*? Marty believed you could, and he went so far as to launch a blind prospective study involving women subjected to the investigation of a breast nodule. His hypothesis was the following: the more defective the mentalisation, the higher the risk of finding a malignant nodule. I must acknowledge my reservations regarding this form of research, which seems to raise a variety of issues. First of all, it goes hand in hand with a kind of medicalisation, which is at odds with the psychoanalytic approach, insofar as it assumes that the investigation brings together an 'objective' observer on the one hand and an objectified patient on the other. Besides, the two clinical situations that serve as a starting point to this volume show us how complex things actually are. Granted, Cate seems to have fewer inner resources available to her than Jasmine: she is more prone to immediate action and agitation as a defence against a constant threat of breakdown. But the narcissistic wound that Jasmine suffers from, while overlaid with an apparently neurotic functioning, is not less deep and might shield a more serious form of disorganisation. In other words, and as Freud points out in relation to fetishism (Freud, 1927), we must often content ourselves with exploring how things have developed following a certain direction (towards fetishism as opposed to a neurotic development, or towards a serious somatisation as opposed to reversible illnesses), without being able to explain why events took this turn as opposed to that one.

That said, the heuristic value of the model of psychosomatic investigation remains in my view. Contrary to Cremerius, quoted by Eva, I do not think that operative functioning should only be seen as an artificial result of the investigations implemented at the Paris Psychosomatic Institute. I believe that operative thinking refers to modalities of drive-related extinction, which can assume a very general form and be regularly found. In other words, I think we do complete a first stage of investigation in which we strive to grasp the strengths and weaknesses of our interlocutor's functioning before we embark on a treatment which will be informed by such strengths and weaknesses.

However, I would like to make two major amendments to the classical Paris School model. First of all, I think we should pay less attention to the notions of preconscious functioning and structure in favour of a focus on elements which, in initial meetings, can alert an attentive and open-minded analyst to the presence of early narcissistic wounds and to the enmeshment of narcissistic and erotic issues. As Marina Perris-Myttas rightly stresses, and as Fotis Bobos shows in another register, such wounds could in fact lead to a somatic outcome. Second, and most importantly, only the analyst's ability to sense the spectral presence of these elements hovering over the first sessions will enable a change in the course of these treatments, turning such wounds into pivotal moments of investigation. This state of affairs is evidenced in both Cate's and Jasmine's cases. If Marina had not been alerted to the overly direct and non-conflicted aspect of her patient's wish for analysis, the situation could have easily evolved into an analysis of the neurotic surface in which everybody is content, but nothing ever happens. Fotis's patient also illustrates this stunningly: the first meeting with her analyst was within a hair's breadth of not happening, and we do not know who, out of the two potential partners, acted out the non-meeting with the object that constituted such a key hurdle in this woman's history: did the analyst fail to hear the doorbell, already caught up in some negative pre-countertransference, or was the patient bound up in the repetition compulsion beyond the pleasure principle?

In other words, the analyst's countertransferential involvement plays a key role in these investigations. As a result, we step outside a purely diagnostical perspective and distance ourselves from the medical dimension of Marty's model. More specifically, we should understand the diagnostic perspective as embedded in the play of transference and countertransference from the outset, which mobilises in the analyst the most archaic aspects of his or her functioning. Here, and more than ever, the importance of the analyst's analysis – or analyses – is absolutely decisive. To put it in a nutshell, we shift from the classical psychosomatic investigation (which consists in an investigation *of the patient*) to the psychosomatic investigation of the *analytic couple* and of *the transferential/countertransferential dynamics* as they are played out in the very first meetings, sometimes even before.

Therefore, I would like to place at the heart of the psychosomatic investigation what I see as a key dialectic. On the one hand, the investigation requires an objectifying impulse that grasps the strong points and weak points of the patient's functioning. And on the other hand, it requires paying attention to the way the patient's strengths and weaknesses play themselves out, often through action, in the very first exchanges between the patient and the analyst. Exploring this dialectic in a creative way, and not obliterating either of the two poles, is in my view at the core of the analytic work with psychosomatic patients. While this applies to the early psychosomatic investigation, it also informs the subsequent treatment, as we are about to see.

The course of treatment

As I mentioned, Marty coined the phrase 'maternal function' to describe the role of the analyst working with severely somatising patients. Let us be clear, the point is not to mother patients, but to protect them against a surplus of excitation that they are not in a position to metabolise, and – Marty insisted on this a lot – to stimulate them enough, especially by reviving their associative and thought processes. In *L'ordre psychosomatique*, Marty devotes a whole chapter to this notion, insisting on the mother's ability to identify with the needs of her child immediately and with no secondarisation (Marty, 1980, pp. 36–37). Despite the differences in theoretical frameworks, and even though in the rest of Marty's book more emphasis is laid on a much more classical approach, Winnicott's primary maternal preoccupation naturally comes to mind (Winnicott, 1956). In my view, at the time that Marty was writing, he lacked the clinical and theoretical tools to tackle these aspects of the transference and countertransference – aspects which, in the aftermath of Winnicott and Bion's work, have taken on such importance in contemporary psychoanalysis over the past thirty years.

On a related note, Marty argued that the presence of a serious somatic illness unconditionally ruled out the possibility of a classical analysis on the couch and required face-to-face treatment with relatively low frequency (once weekly, sometimes twice weekly). This perspective is now out of date for two reasons. Besides the by now obsolete idea that psychoanalysis lacks the tools required to tackle the type of functioning at work in the patients discussed here, let us add another fact; Marty developed his psychoanalytic activity in France in the 1950s and 1960s where he repeatedly witnessed the disasters, including somatic ones, that can ensue when analysts hold neurosis as their sole reference, and are unable to hear the narcissistic suffering veiled by the neurotic element. Fortunately, things have changed, bringing me back to the point of view I just put forward regarding the investigation: the analyst's own analysis – or analyses – is the decisive factor. Analysts who are able to tackle narcissistic wounds in their own personal development will be in a position to face their patients' narcissism; their negative capability (Bion) will make them apt companions along the way, leading them to confront the echo of a Winnicottian breakdown that often dwells at the heart of these treatments, as seen in the two clinical cases discussed: Jasmine tries to keep this threat under control by suppressing her drive-related motions, while Cate strives to escape from it through a disorganised hyperactivity akin to manic defence.

A good ear for the threat of breakdown does not mean overlooking the sexual and erotic factors, quite the opposite; the enmeshment of both these registers is illustrated most strikingly in Jasmine's case. More specifically, it is the analysis of this enmeshment that yields a mutative change;[2] long is the path leading to the possibility of the analyst's interpretation of, and the patient's ability to hear, the intensity of the erotic desire (being seen naked in her nightgown), even though this also refers to a traumatic situation – exposing her genitals to her cousin who looks at her and turns away. Only *after* this desire has been accessed do the analytic couple arrive at the underlying narcissistic wound – the fact of not having been seen by her mother. Such a sequence is exemplary. The point is never to let go of either of these two threads or their moving, yet permanent, entanglement.

I would like to make one last comment in relation to Jasmine's case. While it is true that we no longer hesitate to take on somatising patients in analysis, it nonetheless remains important to be ready to face the emergence of somatic manifestations in the course of these treatments. Some are relatively benign, such as tinnitus, hypertension or tachycardia. Others – such as breast cysts – can conversely lead the analyst to face his or her limits. Taking the weight of external reality into account without ever stopping to be an analyst *and* assuming an inevitable sense of guilt ('does the analysis have anything to do with it?') without lapsing into negative megalomania ('it's all my fault, I did everything wrong'), such are the most daunting clinical tasks at play in these situations.

Commentary

CHRISTIAN SEULIN

The two authors have numerous points of convergence in their reflections on the technical issues of the psychosomatic approach. They agree on questioning the theoretical and technical positions of the Paris Psychosomatic School, especially Marty's contributions, in light of the evolution of contemporary psychoanalytic thought.

The investigation

Eva Schmid-Gloor refers to the work of Cremerius, a German psychoanalyst who puts forward the hypothesis that Marty's account of operative thinking was artificial because of the conditions in which his meetings with patients were held. Jacques Press makes a case for the importance of locating narcissistic deficiencies, which are much more significant in his view than the question of the depth of the preconscious. But more importantly, the transferential-countertransferential dynamic is what should vitally be grasped in the course of the investigation. Both authors indeed emphasise the prominent place occupied by the countertransference in the assessment of the meeting and the somatic risk. We might want to question the terms transference and countertransference in the context of the initial meetings of the investigation. I tend to consider that, while the patient may develop certain modalities of investment in the meeting, it is certainly a bit premature to speak of transference at this stage. In the analyst, conversely, who has experience of psychoanalytic meetings and treatments, the term countertransference seems justified insofar as the analyst's countertransference precedes the patient's transference, as shown by Michel Neyraut (Neyraut, 1974). Sharpened by the analyst's own experience of analysis, the countertransference is a therapeutic tool mobilised in the observation and treatment of the patient. This countertransferential tool is all the more discriminating, as the analyst will have encountered archaic registers beyond neurotic anxieties and conflicts in his or her analyses.

Eva and Jacques link together narcissistic deficiencies, which could be described as identity or borderline identity narcissistic disorders, with the risk of somatisation. As Eva underlines, this point has also arisen in our working group, where not all the members are experienced in psychosomatics, but all are accustomed to the treatment of patients referred to as borderline. We should think of borderline more as clinical situations defined in time and space than rigid states, for we know how heterogeneous the functioning of each patient can be. I will add, following Roussillon, that what is at stake is more likely to pertain to the question of borderline situations in the analysis (Roussillon, 1991). This includes the possibility of a borderline functioning that has so far gone unnoticed, or that has been triggered by internal or environmental changes.

I would happily endorse Jacques' suggestion about the initial meetings and investigation that what is important is the tension between the objectifying account of the patient's narcissistic deficiencies and their enactment in the initial contact. What is important is the psychosomatic investigation of the analytic couple and of the transference-countertransference factors. From my point of view, each human being consists in a psychosomatic unit, and with every patient I see, I pay special attention to the somatic manifestations during the consultation with a view to assessing the somatic risk.

The progress of the treatment

A key question is whether there exists a relevant frame and technique for dealing with somatising patients. Both authors question the absolute validity of the model involving infrequent and face-to-face sessions, as advocated by the Paris Psychosomatic School. Indeed, in our group especially, some analysts work with somatic patients in the framework of frequent sessions on the couch. Of utmost importance is the assessment of areas of narcissistic fragility in connection with traumas; this will influence the analyst's decision regarding the modalities of treatment. Indeed, some instances of destabilising psychic mobilisation may contribute to a somatic accident. Eva thinks that all the cases studied in our working group exemplify a link between the initial meeting and the subsequent development of the analytic process.

Jacques offers to revisit Marty's long-established point that the analyst of psychosomatic patients assumes a maternal function in the transference, expanding this idea in relation to the contributions of Bion and Winnicott whose theoretical advances led to technical improvements. Another factor plays an important role: nowadays, in their personal analysis, analysts explore aspects that go far beyond the oedipal register. This makes them more able to use their countertransference and face the enmeshment of narcissistic and erotic issues when they work with their patients. An important aspect underlined by both authors is sensitivity to the patient's risk of somatisation in the course of the treatment, bearing in mind that a human being is a psychosomatic whole and that no one is omnipotent in his or her prognosis or responsibilities when a somatic issue arises.

Eva offers a detailed discussion of the analytic treatment, on the couch, of Jasmine who combines functional symptoms of symbolic value with other symptoms that show the vestiges of early trauma in the maternal relationship, which will become symbolised via the elaboration of the countertransference, leading to a meaningful transformation. The expression of the patient's trauma is primarily pre-verbal. The analyst must assume the position of the deficient primary object in her countertransference; she must tolerate formlessness without overlooking the erotic dimension. A parallel can be drawn with the treatment of borderline patients in which we also encounter the splitting off of non-symbolised archaic experiences.

Cate's major breakdown and serious somatic illness have an immediate impact on the analyst's countertransference, leading to a face-to-face treatment dotted with pitfalls. At bottom, the questions of the choice of setting and way to conduct the treatment are complex. They involve an assessment of the severity of the narcissistic deficiencies at play, and of the types of intervention-interpretation, and anaclisis or leaning-on, which are desirable in the intersubjective dynamic of the analytic couple; the assessment should reflect a quest for optimum attunement to the patient's needs. I personally think that only a case by case approach should determine the choice of treatment, whether this pertains to the setting or frequency of sessions, and this should put into question an objectifying perspective likely to be too systematic or categorical.

Notes

1 This statement must be qualified. It reflects Marty's position regarding severe illnesses, what he refers to as 'disorganisations' (cancers and auto-immune diseases). Conversely, his perspective was much more nuanced regarding illnesses with critical characteristics (allergies, migraines, etc.).

2 I develop this aspect in more detail in Chapter 1, 'Depression and psychosomatics'.

References

Cremerius, J. (1977) 'Ist die "psychosomatische Struktur" der französischen Schule krankheitsspezifisch?', *Psych–Z. Psychoanaly* 31, 4, pp. 293–317. Stuttgart: Klett-Cotta Verlag.

Freud, S. (1927) *Fetishism*, in *S.E., Vol. 21*. London: The Hogarth Press, pp. 152–58.

Marty, P. (1980) *L'ordre psychosomatique*. Paris: Payot.

Marty, P., de M'Uzan, M. and David, C. (1962) *L'investigation psychosomatique*. Paris: Presses Universitaires de France.

Neyraut, M. (1974) *Le transfert*. Paris: Presses Universitaires de France.

Press, J. (2016) 'Metapsychological and clinical issues in psychosomatics research', *Int. J. Psychoanal.*, 97, pp. 89–113.

Roussillon, R. (1991) *Paradoxes et situations limites de la psychanalyse*. Paris: Presses Universitaires de France.

Winnicott, D.W. (1956) 'Primary Maternal Preoccupation' in *Through Paediatrics to Psycho-analysis*. London: The Hogarth Press, 1975, pp. 278–94.

Chapter 5

Transference and countertransference

MARINA PERRIS-MYTTAS

In 1974, Michel Neyraut suggested that the concept of transference appears *après-coup* in Freud's early work. Transference is seen by Freud, Neyraut suggests, as 'preceded by something' (Neyraut, 2010, p. 218). Furthermore, Neyraut continues, 'it is not only second in the history of analytic thought, it also appears to come second in the analytic treatments' (2010, p. 218) In what follows, drawing from the material of the two clinical cases, I will examine the interplay between the transference and countertransference when working with patients with physical illnesses.

Initial consultations

In both cases discussed in the clinical chapters, it is the analyst's countertransference that first enters the analytic scene. Cate's analyst first encounters his patient through a message left on his answering machine: a woman who speaks in a pressurised way asks for an appointment. She says she wants to have psychotherapy 'for a short while'. Her request evokes in the analyst 'an unpleasant feeling, a negative countertransferential mood', since she does not offer to become a long-term psychoanalytic patient, which her analyst would have wanted. The analyst's negative reaction is accentuated when, in the recorded message, he hears something that sounds like a man's first name in the way the patient identifies herself. Our introduction to the first analytic encounter takes place through the analyst's countertransference. The opening of the analytic work with Jasmine is similar. The most salient feature of the two initial interviews is the analyst's reaction: the analyst is invaded by the clamorous question, 'what does this articulate, thoughtful woman needs analysis for?' The analyst's attempt to focus her analytic listening and attention on the patient is interrupted by this intrusive question, and she is left feeling troubled and confused.

The initial consultations with these two patients brought to mind Bion's notion of an 'emotional storm', a notion which I believe its rooted in Freud's proposition that 'it is a most remarkable thing that the unconscious of one human being can react upon that of another, without passing through the Cs' (Freud, 1915, p. 194). In a similar manner, for Bion the 'emotional storm' is to be expected when 'two personalities meet' (Bion, 1979, p. 247). It seems to me that this storm comes into being as the winds of unconscious communication between the two protagonists gathers force and intensity. With both patients, the 'storm' of the initial encounter rages in the analysts. With Cate, the storm is initiated before her actual arrival through her request that her therapy lasts 'a short while'. She arrives for her session, she leaves, and she returns. All of this before she actually meets her analyst to be. Is all this movement a sign of enacted transference? In the actual session there is no sign of emotional turbulence in the patient. Whatever turbulence is present is felt by the analyst.

In Jasmine's initial consultations, psychic unrest is even more concealed, to both herself and to the analyst. The 'storm' is barely discernible in her, but it is, as we have seen, very present in the analyst's countertransference. When she finds herself in less treacherous weather, the analyst observes these stormy countertransference reactions. Her observations become cornerstones for building her initial response to Jasmine's psychic world. Making use of the countertransference reactions as a compass to navigate the start of the analytic journey is never more important than when working with patients who, like Cate and Jasmine, have a psychosomatic tendency to 'resort' to physical illness. Indeed, for both these patients, it is the analyst's countertransference reactions which seem to have initiated the analytic process.

Marilia Aisenstein has developed this observation further when she points out that in the area of psychosomatics 'the countertransference, or rather what I will call today the co-transference, is at the centre of the co-creation by two psyches that constitutes the psychoanalytic treatment', adding that, 'this is true for all patients, but even more so for patients suffering from somatic illnesses' (Aisenstein, 2013, p. 351).

The centrality of the countertransference

As is well-known, 'countertransference' is a term coined by Freud in 1910 to describe the feelings that arise in the analyst 'as a result of the patient's influence on his unconscious' (Freud, 1910, p. 144). In 1912 in the aftermath of Jung's analysis of Sabina Spielrein, Freud stressed that a 'paper on countertransference is sorely needed' (McGuire, 1974, p. 475). This 'sorely needed' paper was not to be written by Freud. But as psychoanalysis grew and developed over the next century, the interest in the countertransference gathered momentum on both sides of the Atlantic, coming into its own in the 1950s until the present day.

It was Heinrich Racker who, in 1948, building on Freud's notion that the analyst's unconscious understands that of his patient, was the first to suggest that 'countertransference reactions can provide evidence to the analyst of what is going on in the analysand' (Racker, 1948). Soon after, in 1950, we have the arrival of a couple of seminal papers by Paula Heimann and Racker. Both these papers focus on the part played by the patients' projections in the creation of the analyst's countertransference. Furthermore, I cannot stress enough that both Heimann and Racker emphasise that countertransference is only partially the result of the patient's projections. To my mind, this caution is essential for the countertransference to indeed become the powerful tool it can prove to be in helping us find our bearings within the patients' psychic reality.

A few years after Heimann and Racker, in 1952 in France Marty drew attention to the 'difficulty' that psychoanalysts experienced when working with physically ill patients because of the strong countertransference reactions. Aisenstein summarises Marty's observation as follows:

A twofold identificatory process develops in the latter [the analyst]; on the one hand, he experiences personally, through the identification with his patient, the fragmentation of his body and the alteration of his image; and on the other he is subjected to a movement of identification on the patient's part that attacks the quality of the psychoanalyst as object, and thus undermines his sense of alterity or otherness (Aisenstein, 2013, p. 334).

The shifting texture of the transference

I shall now turn my attention to the characteristics of the transference during the phases of somatisation by focusing on two moments in Jasmine's analysis. The first moment, which I shall briefly describe, is that of Jasmine's initial transference response: its *explicit* absence in the two first consultations. The second moment, or period rather, which I shall discuss in some detail, is the opening phase of my patient's physical illness which developed later, a few years into her analysis.

Jasmine did not present with somatic symptoms. Her sudden illness, described in the clinical chapter, occurred just before the analysis was due to start, and came as a surprise to us both. As mentioned above, the 'emotional storm' that Bion would expect to find in an initial consultation, was not discernible in the transference. The early signs of instinctual impulses orienting themselves towards the analyst, the kind of movement we can expect to find in the adequately mentalised neurotic patient, the movement which, with time, forms the transference in its classical sense, was absent in Jasmine. Instead, the first transference response had the quality of an undifferentiated, massive cathexis of the analyst, the sort that Aisenstein considers to be typically present in psychosomatic patients (Aisenstein and Aisemberg, 2010, p. 58). Jasmine said to her analyst 'I like you and I want to work with you'. In my opinion, this initial response was the precursor of the idealisation, blind to the object as such, which fully thrived in later years and became erotised before the period of somatisation.

The second moment to which I will now turn my attention came about a few years into the analysis, and initiated, I believe, Jasmine's somatisation. For a long time, the idealisation of the analyst kept at bay powerful transference longings for an object, her analyst, who was unconsciously experienced as rejecting her and her sexualised need to be taken in. This powerful idealisation – rooted as it was in the projection of her ideal ego, heir of primary narcissistic omnipotence – had acted to a large extent as an obstacle to the gathering of powerful drive forces, both libidinal and aggressive, in fully forming the transference.

In the period preceding the somatisation, and as the exploration of the idealisation became more possible, the intensity and quantity of Jasmine's mute feelings, erotic longings par excellence, towards her object/analyst who she unconsciously experienced as rejecting, overwhelmed any capacity for psychic elaboration she had developed during the years of analysis. At this juncture, gradually and steadily the analyst witnessed an apparent disappearance of the transference and the development of somatic symptoms.

André Green describes the transference as:

> . . . the lever of psychoanalytic action, its essential given, which involves – beyond the affect-representation division – the incitement to movement of psychical activity that cathects an unconscious object, and allows contact between the traces left by objects from the past and the new object of the analytic situation in a new and original formulation.
>
> (Green, 2005, p. 260)

It was this *levering* function of the transference, albeit compromised by this powerful idealisation, which seems to have been lost at the moment of somatisation. Instead of developing transference feelings, the analytic scene was filled with a pervasive, diffuse anxiety. Whatever the communication was at that time it was unintelligible, and it started to unfold in action: not an acting out but an acting-in the body which followed the path of a 'somatic regression'.

'Somatic regression', a term developed by the Paris School of Psychosomatics (Smadja, 2005, p. 31), is an instance of what Freud identified as the 'mysterious leap' – 'a process in which the mental apparatus switches off'. It is considered to be reversible. 'The somatic reaction has kicked in, more or less totally, substituting for the psychical reaction' (Smadja, 2005, p. 32). With the advent of the somatic regression, the *levering* function of the transference is undone, causing the transference to assume a different texture.

Up until the appearance of physical symptoms, Jasmine's transference developed to a great extent under the sway of the pleasure principle (albeit infiltrated with strong narcissistic features) and could therefore function as a lever in the analytic work. I want to suggest that with the advent of somatisation, a powerful quantity of the destructive drive Thanatos began to dominate in the alloy of Eros and Thanatos. As the drive movement – or rather the movement of the alloy of Eros and Thanatos – was diverted to its somatic origin, the transference began to lack its characteristic quality of mobility and displacement; as a consequence, it lost its levering function. Instead, the analysis was flooded by the inertia characteristic of the repetition compulsion, and the transference acquired a texture marked by the absence of specific qualified affects, which were transformed to a diffuse and pervasive anxiety.

Transference and countertransference develop in tandem, each prompting the other. And often, as we saw with Jasmine (Section I) in the development of the last cyst in her breast, the work in the countertransference potentiates the transference's return to its levering function. One last point on the countertransference when working with patients who somatise – we often see that the countertransference is first experienced by the analyst at a somatic level (Perris, 2017).

The emergence of the entwined transference and the countertransference confronts us, even more acutely when experienced on the somatic level, with an ever-present conundrum: what part of the analyst's reaction results from the patient's unconscious communication, and what comes from the analyst's own transference to the analysand? Indeed, in considering the interconnection of the transference and countertransference, it is crucial to take note of Racker's and Heimann's warning that the analyst distinguish between countertransference feelings arising from projection and those arising from their own transference to the patient. For the most part, the differentiation may be very hard to achieve, but I think the attempt to make the distinction must still be our aim.

End thoughts

By way of closure I want to return to the clinical picture. In Section I, in the detailed sessional material, we saw that Jasmine's analyst interpreted the patient's nascent desire to be looked at and touched by the analyst. With hindsight, this interpretation can be seen to be rather premature, as the erotic transference was still repressed and distant from the patient's awareness. Nevertheless, through the analysis of the dream which was brought in the session that followed, the analyst arrived at the image of the baby at the breast enjoying the moment of blissful satisfaction. She felt a 'strong aversion to the scene'. Something of traumatic intensity was occurring: the impact of an early trauma appeared in the analytic scene in its current version. In the days that followed, the analyst and the patient arrived at a construction of the mother's difficulties (her strong aversion) in allowing herself to 'be used as a receptacle' for her infant's instinctual life.

Jasmine's overly anxious mother (anxious about her own sexuality) had a traumatic impact on Jasmine. The intensity of uncontained bodily excitation in her mother's arms left in its wake representational gaps and a seriously compromised capacity for communicating her own eroticism to her object. In her analysis, under the sway of the transference, split-off early experiences of trauma that stemmed from the era of primary narcissism returned and could be worked through. In bringing my remarks to a close, I want to stress the importance of two transformational moments. In the first instance, as there were no words for these experiences, they were 'spoken' in the language of the body. That is, they were articulated through the body via the emergence of somatic symptoms. A second transformation took place through the activation of the analyst's countertransference. In the sessions that followed, through the trajectory of the movements in the transference and the countertransference, an opening was created in the analytic process, which led to the beginnings of containment of excess affectivity and allowed for the qualification of the affect anxiety. The transference affects acquired depth and could eventually be revealed, while the transference regained its leverage function.

EVA SCHMID-GLOOR

Transference and countertransference in psychosomatics pose a particular challenge. For the Paris School of Psychosomatics (Pierre Marty, Michel de M'Uzan, Marilia Aisenstein, Claude Smadja, and others), the psychosomatic individual appears to function in a concrete way, presenting 'operative thinking' – the lack of a capacity to elaborate and mentalise by representations. According to Marty, this psychic functioning stems from a state of negativity, which is the outcome of a disorganisation process. And it is this state of negativity that Marty associates with a life characterised by a relentless movement that proceeds in the direction of undoing psychic meaning and complexity.

As has become clear from the various discussions, all of the members of our Working Group on Psychosomatics subscribed to the view that there was sufficient evidence to believe that the majority of the psychosomatic patients are, in effect, taken over by a state of negativity. Discussing this issue further, we would then come up with a number of questions such as: are we able to make out or construct in the *après-coup* of an ongoing analysis what in the patient's past has led to an implicit disorganisation process linked to a somatic crisis? Or do certain psychosomatic symptoms represent at a very archaic primary level some symbolic meaning? (A position most of the authors would disagree with). Or are these symptoms rather – as most of the authors would claim – devoid of any symbolic meaning, which implies that meaning only can result from a retrospective construction?

These questions also become relevant when considering the issue of *transference and countertransference* in psychosomatics. Working at deeper levels with our patients, we inevitably come into touch with traces of undone or unlived life, which can be related to archaic states of mind. We then may speculate – although many of the theoreticians would object to this idea – about the possibility of receiving messages on a more bodily, sensorial level, which might be contained in the psychosomatic symptom. A way of *thinking with the body* would then become a crucial tool for treating psychosomatic patients. All of this is a point of departure for the possible work of transformation in the transference and countertransference. I would argue that we should give room for the idea of thinking about different forms and levels of symbolic functioning, rather than speaking in terms of either the absence or presence of symbolic functioning.

During the past few years in psychoanalytic publications on the topic of psychosomatics, there appear to be two schools of thought around the origin, development, and treatment of psychosomatic symptoms (Gubb, 2013). The first, as we have seen, is the well-established Paris School of Psychosomatics, which has put forward the most coherent and well-developed psychoanalytic theorisation of the topic of psychosomatics to this day. The second approach does not formally exist but is commonly referred to as the attachment approach, since there are a number of authors who theorise about the treatment of psychosomatic symptoms from the perspective of attachment theory, and who stress the importance of the quality of the object for the structuring of the drives. The way in which problems of mentalisation are linked to psychosomatic illness is conceived by the Paris School of Psychosomatics as the 'speechless mind' and by the attachment school as the 'communicating body' (Gubb, 2013).

Several authors (Taylor, Sloate, Griffies, and Katz among them) believe that the mothers of psychosomatic patients were unable to attune to their infant, and thus failed to regulate and organise the child's experiences, as a consequence, the infant was not able to develop a capacity to modulate its own arousal of archaic sensations and other affective states of excitation or overstimulation. Psychosomatic patients often describe their mothers as being either over-possessive or overwhelming or unattuned to the needs of their child. Such a mother may have engaged with her child's body as though it was her own narcissistic possession, i.e. some kind of self-object, and therefore some authors describe the experience of having 'one body for two' (e.g. Taylor, 2008). In order to function, the child may develop a split in his or her ego, which will create a picture of pseudo-normal robot-like functioning. Referring to such patients, Gérard Szwec coined the phrase 'the willing galley slaves' (Szwec, 1998).

Many of these patients can achieve great success in isolated areas of their lives; however, in creating this split, their archaic and unprocessed affects, particularly those regarding separation, remain unintegrated and unsymbolised. And it is thus the working-through of this split that has to take a central role in the analysis in the transference-countertransference interplay. My own clinical experience with psychosomatic patients (and not only with them) brought me to realise that finding a way to listen to the *'speaking body'* – be it the patient's or the analyst's one – might become one of the crucial tools for our clinical work.

The German psychoanalyst Jörg Scharff criticises the attitude of analysts who, concerning the patient-analyst relationship, 'all-too-soon deflect their attention from the corporeal aspects and from the awareness of the immediate and continual reciprocal impact upon each other, in order to rather resort to the world of the imaginary and the *reifying thinking*, cut off from the workings of the body' (Scharff, 2010, p. 10). He emphasises that only through the immediate experience of our sensory perceptions can analysts be open to the unconscious, and so he is in favour of the analyst carefully listening to the interplay of sensory perceptions and reverie. He writes:

> In sensing and listening to our corporeal responsiveness to the patient's state of mind and corporeal being, we let ourselves be seized by the situation as it evolves between analyst and patient, not unlike when we commit and dedicate ourselves to a work of art.
>
> (Scharff, 2010, p. 11)

In this context, Scharff speaks of a 'pre-reflexive sensory interrelation' of the analyst's and analysand's 'bodily presence' (Scharff, 2010, p. 14) which, as I view it, particularly come into effect in the transference-countertransference processes in the treatment of the psychosomatic patient. Yet to engage with the patient on such a profound and fundamental level brings us in close contact with the most intimate and precarious parts of ourselves, which we may not be prepared and willing to do, not least because we may fear that the highly valued flow of ideas and thoughts that we commonly rely upon so much, may be interrupted and get out of control. So, I would say that it is no wonder we are inclined to cling on to theoretical considerations rather than open up and emotionally resonate with the constant state of physical and mental pain and suffering that some of our patients confront us with, and which inevitably place a huge strain on the analyst.

In order to support this line of argumentation I am now going to present a clinical example taken from the treatment of one of my patients, which has had a profound effect on me. From the beginning of Paolo's analysis, I had to make huge efforts of psychical and mental work on a pre-symbolic and corporeal-sensory level to get the analysis off the ground. Paolo had an extremely difficult infancy and childhood with an over-stimulating mother and an explosive and chaotic father. Already as an infant he recurrently fell ill with several life-threatening diseases, so that during infancy he only narrowly escaped from dying of meningitis and pneumonia. During his adolescence most of his psychic problems were seemingly solved mainly by his extraordinary artistic talent, opening the way for artistic sublimation. And eventually Paolo was even considered to be an infant prodigy. He could invest a huge amount of drive energy in his artistic work as a painter. The sublimated, highly educated part of Paolo became split off from another archaic, chaotic and raw part of him, which insisted on immediate drive satisfaction. A part which during analysis we aimed to link with meaning and to integrate.

During the initial phase of his analysis, Paolo recurrently came down with one or other infectious diseases, especially during the holiday breaks when I wasn't present. At a later phase of his analysis, the *raw part* of his psychic life would make itself *heard* and instead of the earlier *acting-ins* in the body, we saw an increasing number of *acting outs*. This was actually the time when his somatisation disorders stopped.

In his transference Paolo would experience me in two ways: When I held on to the basic payment rule, I became icy cold; when for a specific reason I once offered him a session time that suited him better, I became an incestuous seductress. Theoretically, I understood this as a transference situation with the early mother. We talked in great length about the double-bind he put me in by experiencing me as ice-cold or dangerously seductive, with no space for anything else. Yet in the end it became clear that he was completely unable to make use of what we understood cognitively and we found ourselves blocked.

So I decided to discuss the case with a group of colleagues. I spoke to them about my intense countertransference feelings in a hopeless situation, where I had the impression that I could not do anything right by my patient, which left me feeling paralysed and numb. After a while, one of the colleagues said that within the last few minutes he had started to feel physically quite awful, he felt so constricted as if he was being suffocated. And he strongly suspected that his feelings had something to do with the clinical situation I just had described. What this colleague described made me immediately think of the bodily sensations Paolo experienced in his childhood: when he felt uncontained by his environment and feared catastrophe, he would sometimes psychically shut himself off, and become paralysed.

I could for the first time conceive of my bodily countertransference feelings as being a response to the imminent, underlying bodily sensations of my patient, and now I was able to talk to Paolo and let him know that I had understood how paralysed and imprisoned he must have felt as a boy when he was terribly afraid of being alive and moving around freely, and had to control himself powerfully because he felt unprotected and lacking any secure hold from his environment. Paolo sighed and showed relief when he realised he had reached me on this fundamental level. This interpretation of my countertransference obviously needed the triangular situation with the colleague who was capable of receiving Paolo's bodily message as a third person.

Only after Paolo experienced his yearning to be being held in the transference situation could he recognise that his self-holding had always been a suffocating self-imprisonment, an inner state, which had directly impacted upon me in the analytic situation. So, when I was finally able to listen to my own bodily feelings of self-imprisonment and self-constriction, I could open up to his yearning to be held. Consequently, in some brief moments Paolo could allow himself to experience certain more or less explosive drive-related impulses, and he could also realise how much he wanted to possess, dominate and penetrate me.

Whereas my countertransference concerned essentially an identificatory level with my patient's early experiences, with Marina Perris, her countertransference concerned the inner object of her patient – her 'inner mother'. In that sense my countertransference corresponds to what Heinrich Racker calls a 'concordant identification' (identification of the analyst with the ego and the id of the patient), and Marina's countertransference is linked more to a 'complementary identification' (identification with the inner objects of the patient) (Racker, 1950).

Coming back to my patient, I would like to finish by noting that while other patients might find stability and refuge in self-calming rituals, perverse activities, or taking addictive drugs, from adolescence onwards Paolo had chosen a path of partial *over-sublimation*. He had to pay a price for this: his psychosomatic fragility persisted into adolescence and early adulthood, and in times of the merest psychic stress he still was prone to fall ill. I think it was due to his sublimatory activity that Paolo was not entirely cut off from the work of drive transformation, albeit his artistic activities revealed certain features similar to those mechanical, self-calming rituals employed by other patients. When in the beginning of his analysis Paolo described his way of painting it reminded me more of the self-calming rituals (*autocalmants*) described by Gérard Szwec (Szwec, 1998) than a sublimatory activity. For hours on end Paolo would indulge in mechanically painting geometric forms while simultaneously watching television programmes. Describing patients who resort to mechanical self-calming rituals devoid of auto-erotic qualities for the purpose of discharging excitation, Szwec refers to extreme athletes who manage to repress one type of excitation by producing another. It occurred to me that Paolo's artistic practice served a similar function to the mechanical self-calming rituals described by Szwec.

Szwec describes babies with non-responsive mothers who achieve premature autonomy by seeking refuge in self-calming rituals. By transforming themselves into mechanical cradling machines, these babies make a desperate attempt to fend off the representational void that comes from the failure of a good enough holding maternal object. The mechanical self-calming ritual can be seen as an emergency attempt to bind the libidinally unbound death drive, and achieve a better fusion of the drives, which mental activity had not been able to accomplish.

Commentary

LUIGI SOLANO

My overriding impression is that Marina Perris and Eva Schmid-Gloor focus on two different aspects of the transference and countertransference, but their positions are generally compatible and complementary; the two different aspects, as outlined by Eva, are on the one hand, a 'speechless mind' and on the other, a 'communicating body'. Eva explores the 'communicating body', starting with the possibility of receiving messages on a bodily, sensorial level, and consequently expressing communications at that level. Her idea of countertransference is a way of 'thinking with the body' in the interplay of somatic sensations and reverie that 'can become a crucial tool for treating psychosomatic patients'. At this point we can see at play both a somatic transference and a somatic countertransference: finding a way to listen to the 'communicating body' – be it the patient's or the analyst's one – may be one of the crucial tools for our clinical work.[1]

Scharff's work (2010) is quoted by Eva Schmid-Gloor in connection with what I would call the importance of remaining at a bodily level with the patient.[2] He speaks of 'sensing and listening to our corporeal responsiveness to the patient's state of mind and corporeal being', of a 'pre-reflexive sensory interrelation' of the analyst's and analysand's 'bodily presence'. This bodily aspect is based on 'early sensory experiences and feelings of infantile object-relatedness'. Contact with this dimension allows the analyst to get in touch with parts of the patient that were split off in response to a narcissistic way of caregiving; the transference-countertransference interplay at this bodily level may succeed in working through this split. Eva is well aware of the difficulties of this contact, which involve, 'the most intimate and precarious parts of our selves'.

Marina seems to focus more on the 'speechless mind' aspect of somatic patients. She begins by noticing how the reports of both clinical cases (Cate and Jasmine) begins with countertransference reactions, which somehow take centre stage, both substituting and indicating the patients' difficulties. These are seen as part of what Bion called 'emotional storm taking place when two personalities meet', following Freud's concept of direct communication between the unconscious of two human beings. In this case the emotional storm appears in the analyst, rather than in the patient.

All this could be brought back by someone to a notion of projective identification, but when looking more closely at the mechanism of projection, Marina is careful to specify (following Heimann, Racker and Aisenstein) that the analyst's countertransference is only partly due to the patient's projections. She also considers the importance of an attempt to differentiate the countertransference feelings arising from projection and those arising from the analyst's own transference to the patient, though this differentiation may never be exhaustive.

In the 'speechless mind' aspect of Marina case, she notes that transference appears absent, at least explicitly, in Jasmine's initial consultations. What may be sensed under this absence is 'an undifferentiated, massive cathexis of the analyst', a precursor of idealisation, blind to the object as such, a projection onto the analyst of the ideal ego of narcissistic omnipotence. At this point, somatic symptoms develop 'when the intensity and quantitative dimension of these mute feelings towards her rejecting object/analyst overwhelmed the capacity for psychic elaboration'. Here, somatic communication appears to emerge as an *effect* of the insufficient work of the preconscious (an effect of the speechless mind). This appears to be different to Eva's formulation, where somatic communication has a form of autonomy and possibly takes place *before* the mind is called upon to operate. Eva states that 'huge efforts of psychical and mental work on a pre-symbolic as well as on a corporeal-sensory level were required' to begin with, and I would stress, before reaching symbolic, mentalised levels. Work on the pre-symbolic level is required in order 'to link with meaning and to integrate' a pre-symbolic part that was originally split off as a response to inadequate holding.

Both authors, on the one hand, make an effort to link their observations with Freud's (second topic) drive theory. Eva speaks of self-calming rituals as having the aim of 'binding the not enough libidinally bound death drive . . . and achieving by this a better fusion of the drives'. Marina expresses her view of Jasmine's onset of somatisation as linked to a prevalence of Thanatos in the alloy of drives, which causes changes in the quality of the transference, suffused with inertia and devoid of its 'levering' function. Both authors, on the other hand, pay great importance to early trauma and the lack of holding/containment as predispositions to the emergence of somatic symptoms and other forms of pathology and as conditioning the development of certain qualities of the transference.

Notes

1 To the authors quoted here who have contributed to work in this field, I would add the work of Italian psychoanalyst Carla De Toffoli (De Toffoli, 2011; 2014), who has introduced impressive clinical examples in these areas.
2 In connection to this I would also quote another Italian colleague, Agostino Racalbuto (Racalbuto, 1994).

References

Aisenstein, M. (2013) 'Transference and countertransference with somatic patients', in *Transference and Countertransference Today*. London: The New Library of Psychoanalysis.
Aisenstein, M. and Aisemberg, E.R. (2010) *Psychosomatics Today: A Psychoanalytical Perspective*. London: Karnac.
Bion, W.R. (1979) 'Making the Best of a Bad Job', in *Clinical Seminars and Four Papers*. Abingdon: Fleetwood Press, 1987.
Britton, R. (2003) *Sex, Death and the Superego: Experiences in Psychoanalysis*. London: Karnac.
De M'Uzan, M. (2013) *Death and Identity: Being and the Psycho-sexual Drama*. London: Karnac.
De Toffoli, C. (2011) 'The living body in the psychoanalytic experience', *Psychoanalytic Quarterly*, 80, pp. 595–618.
De Toffoli, C. (2014) *Transiti corpo-mente: l'esperienza della psicoanalisi* [Body–Mind Transitions: The Psychoanalytic Experience]. Edited by Basilio Bonfiglio. Milan: Franco Angeli.
Freud, S. (1910) *Five Lectures on Psycho-Analysis, Leonardo da Vinci and Other Work*, in *S.E., Vol. 11*. London: The Hogarth Press, 1973.
Freud, S. (1915) 'The Unconscious', in *Papers on Metapsychology, S.E., Vol. 14*. London: The Hogarth Press, 1973.
Freud, S. (1920) *Beyond the Pleasure Principle, Group Psychology and Other Works, S.E., Vol. 18*. London: The Hogarth Press, 1973.
Green, A. (1997) *On Private Madness*. London: Karnac.
Green, A. (2005) *Psychoanalysis: A Paradigm for Clinical Thinking*. Paris: Free Association Books.
Gubb, K. (2013) 'Psychosomatics today: A review of contemporary theory and practice', *Psychoanalytic Review*, 100, pp. 15–165.
Heimann, P. (1950) 'On countertransference', *Int. J. Psychoanal.*, 31, pp. 81–84.
McGuire, W. (1974) *The Freud/Jung Letters*. London: The Hogarth Press and Routledge.
Neyraut, M. (1974) 'Countertransference and psychoanalytic thought', in D. Birksted-Breen, S. Flanders and A. Gibeault (eds), (2010), *Reading French Psychoanalysis*. London: Routledge.
Perris, M. (2017) 'The Soma and the Body: Navigating through the Counter-Transference', British-German Colloquium, Edinburgh.
Racalbuto, A. (1994) *Tra il fare e il dire: L'esperienza dell'inconscio e del non verbale in psicoanalisi* [Between doing and saying: unconscious and non-verbal experience in psychoanalysis]. Milan: Cortina.

Racker, H. (1948) 'A contribution to the problem of countertransference', *Argentine Psychoanalytic Association Meeting*, Buenos Aires, Argentina.
Racker, H. (1950) 'A contribution to the psychoanalysis of transference neurosis', Argentine Psychoanalytic Association Meeting, Buenos Aires, Argentina.
Scharff, J.M. (2010) *Die leibliche Dimension in der Psychoanalyse*. Frankfurt: Brandes & Apsel.
Smadja, C. (2005) *The Psychosomatic Paradox*. London: Free Association Books.
Szwec, G. (1998) *Les galériens volontaires*. Paris: Presses Universitaires de France.
Taylor, G.J. (2008) 'Frontline: Why publish a special issue on psychoanalysis and psychosomatics?', *Journal of the American Academy of Psychoanalysis and Dynamic Psychiatry*, 36, pp. 1–10.

Section IV

Theoretical issues

Chapter 6

Drives and affects

MARINA PERRIS-MYTTAS

During the period of somatisation in Jasmine's analysis, I witnessed her moving away from a self that had previously been alert to her own thoughts, mentations and feelings. Once Jasmine fell ill, she became almost exclusively absorbed with her somatic illnesses. How should we comprehend this transformation? That is the question which I shall address in this chapter.

Early in his work, Freud encountered a similar kind of transformation in patients suffering from hysterical conversion. In 1895 he introduced a metaphor, the 'mysterious leap' (Freud and Breuer, 1895d), to capture the shift he witnessed from the psychic to the somatic. The notion of the 'mysterious leap', which has been subsequently studied and developed by the Paris School of Psychosomatics (Marty, 1958, 1968; Smadja 2005, 2011; Aisenstein 2006, 2010) in their psychoanalytic work with physically ill patients, has proved a pivotal metaphor in the psychoanalytic understanding of psychosomatic illness.

In the course of the analysis of physically ill patients, or when our patients fall physically ill during their analysis, as happened to Jasmine, the conjunction of the mental and the somatic becomes the protagonist of the analytic scene. The study of this conjunction, of which the mysterious leap is one instance, became a central focus of Freud's development of the theory of psychoanalysis. In 1905 in the 'Three Essays on Sexuality', he introduced the concept of the drive as a means of further understanding this conjunction of the somatic and the mental in all its complexity and elusiveness.

On the basis of my clinical experience, I am suggesting that psychoanalytic work with somatic patients offers a privileged vantage point from which to reflect on the centrality of the concept of the drive and its somatic origins, and on the related conceptualisation of the economic dimension in psychoanalytic theory and practice. As described in Section I, during the course of her analysis Jasmine ceased to be the patient she had been for the previous six years, as she became increasingly absorbed by her physical illnesses. What light can the concept of the drive shed on Jasmine's transformation?

In what follows, I will discuss the concept of the drive, particularly in relation to beta elements in Bion's metapsychology. These two concepts have been regarded as having an affinity (Green, 1998; Kohon, 2014; Reed, Levine and Scarfone, 2013; Perris, 2014). I will consider both the extent and the limits of this proposed affinity and I will do so in the context of considering their relative usefulness in grappling with the enigma with which psychosomatic illnesses presents us.

The concept of the drive

As mentioned above, the concept of the drive was first introduced by Freud in 'Three Essays on Sexuality' (Freud, 1905). He returned to the concept ten years later in the first of his *Papers on Metapsychology*, 'Instincts and their Vicissitudes' written in 1915, and he defined the concept as follows:

If now we apply ourselves to considering mental life from a biological point of view, a drive appears to us as a concept on the frontier between the mental and the somatic, as the psychical representative of the stimuli originating from within the organism, and reaching the mind as a measure of the demand made upon the mind for work in consequence of its connection with the body (Freud, 1915, pp. 121–22).

At that time the concept of the drive is explicitly established as a core metapsychological concept. The pressure exercised by the drive, 'its very essence' (1915, p. 122) amounts to the economic aspect which is ubiquitously present in psychic phenomena. When looking at the economic aspect we attempt 'to track the vicissitudes of amounts of excitation and to arrive at least at some relative estimate of their magnitude' (1915, p. 181).

Notwithstanding the problems generated by the choice of the word 'drive' to translate Freud's term *triebe* into English, the concept of the drive, when understood as referring to power and force, is pivotal in psychoanalytic theory and practice. Indeed, it is from this perspective that Freud's notion that affect is 'the exponent of the drive' becomes intelligible, especially when we think of the unremitting force of our patients' affects when they are in the grip of the repetition compulsion.

The drive, as a concept lying on the frontier between the soma and the psyche, has been explored and elaborated by the Paris School of Psychosomatics. They see the concept of the drive and its economic dimension as central to an understanding of somatisation processes. Their clinical and theoretical work has expanded and elucidated Freud's metaphor of the 'mysterious leap' (Freud and Breuer, 1895d), from the body to the mind and vice versa. At the heart of this elaboration is their emphasis on the quantitative dimension of the drive which serves as a bridge to the notion of affect, the 'exponent of the drive'. Andre Green highlights this point clearly and succinctly when he writes that 'the psychical representative of the drive, synonymous with the instinctual impulse, is what will give birth to affect, once the meeting with the object presentation has occurred' (Green, 2005).

To turn to Jasmine, her transformation, as described in Part I, can be seen as an instance of the 'mysterious leap': that of the drive from the psychic to the somatic. From this perspective, the onset of her somatisation occurred at the moment of an excess of drive activity mobilised by intense erotic feelings in the transference which had not achieved psychic representation, could not be psychically elaborated, and in this way they reached a traumatic dimension. The drive regressed to its somatic origins and prompted a physical illness. The unfolding of the analysis of this situation pointed to early maternal traumatism. (For an elaboration of this transformation through the lens of the analytic relationship, see Chapter 5.)

The Freudian drive, Bion's beta elements, the somatic and the psychic

As already mentioned, a number of analytic writers have suggested that Bion's beta elements bear a close affinity with Freud's concept of the drive. What requires further discussion is the nature of this affinity as well as its limits. Exploring the nature of this affinity will hopefully help us to start contemplating whether the concept of beta elements, like the concept of the drive, can offer insight into the process of somatisation.

In tracing Bion's definition of beta elements in the 1960s, we can see that he employs different definitions (Perris, 2014). To summarise, in *Cogitations*, beta elements are pronounced as 'dead, unreal objects' (Bion, 1992), while in *Learning From Experience*, beta elements are defined as 'sense-impressions' (Bion, 1962). In *A Theory of Thinking* they are seen as 'raw-sense' data (Bion, 1962) and in 1963 in *Elements of Psychoanalysis* they are regarded as 'bodily sensations' and later as 'aspects of personality, linked with a sense of catastrophe' (Bion, 1963). To my mind, these different notions of beta elements provoke questions regarding their conceptual specificity and clarity. Indeed, it has been observed that 'Bion's own approach to the subject of definition and nomination was to make a study in its own right even as he used it' (Mawson, 2017, p. 18). Be that as it may, and acknowledging the potential lack of clarity in Bion's definitional accounts, in what follows I will offer some thoughts on the extent of the conceptual affinity between beta elements and the drive.

First, if we were only to focus on the definition of beta elements primarily as 'bodily sensations' (Bion, 1963) we can see that the concept of beta elements is very close to Freud's notion of the drive, in that they both belong to the somatic register. Both concepts seem to be embedded in the same bodily territory of human experience. André Green has emphasised this similarity between the two concepts when he states: 'The id [in Freud's structural model] is made up from impulses, that is a concept that is very close to Bion's b-elements', and he adds, 'He [Bion] is aware of that' (Green, 1998, p. 652).

But also with regard to the limits of this affinity, Green observes that the Freudian drives originate only in the somatic, whereas beta elements do not always originate there. 'The main difference between Bion and Freud', Green suggests, 'could be that for Freud the drives always had their source in the inner part of the body, whereas for Bion b-elements may also arise from external stimuli upon the primordial mind. What is sensuous in the b-elements is more their relationship to the primitive body that lacks a thinker than to the source of the element' (1998, p. 652).

Secondly, when we move from comparing the concepts of drive and beta elements in terms of their origin, to comparing them in relation to the theory of transformation from the somatic to psychic that each implies, we find them to be radically different. For Freud, as for Bion, this transformation is mediated by the primary object, but the process of this transformation is very different in the two. For Freud, the transformation occurs *within the subject*, rather than externally, and the transformation is inherent in the very concept of the drive. From the moment of the baby's *original* 'experience of satisfaction' afforded by the object (Freud, 1900, p. 565), the drive acquires the potential to be constituted in the process of the meeting of the 'demand for work' that the body exerts upon the mind. (Freud, 1915, pp. 121–22), henceforth engendering psychic representations.[1]

For Bion, on the other hand, the subject's beta elements have to be transformed by the object's alpha-function in order to be usable in psychic work. Indeed, without the object's alpha-function, beta elements remain untransformed; they remain b-elements, 'thoughts without a thinker', until such time as the object's reverie will bring about the transformation' (Bion, 1967, p. 116). It is 'the mother's capacity for reverie', Bion continues, which 'is the receptor organ for the infant's harvest of self-sensation gained by its conscious' (Bion, 1962, p. 116).

Thirdly, in my opinion there exists a further source of affinity, as well as of disparity, between the drive and beta elements, which comes from Freud's early work, specifically his 'Project for a Scientific Psychology' in 1895. In this work, Freud identified a process of an amassing of stimuli, an 'accumulation of quantity' *Q* (Freud, 1955 [1895d]) within the mental apparatus. The accrual of stimuli, Freud suggested, can cause an excessive and escalating excitation which burdens the psyche, leading to a primary impulse towards discharge. Such a discharge is required to protect the mental apparatus, which during its early development lacks any protective shield.

As I see it, this notion of an amassing of stimuli, can usefully be seen as the conceptual precursor of both Freud's concept of the drive, as it developed from 1905 in the 'Three Essays on Sexuality' onwards, and of Bion's beta phenomena described in 'A Theory of Thinking' (Bion, 1962). This common ancestry is, I believe, the third element which lies at the root of the affinity between the two concepts. However, as the two concepts evolved out of this common ancestry they followed singular paths, both in their theoretical development and in their clinical implications. For Freud the early notion of accretions of stimuli necessitating their discharge was the precursor of the core concept of his metapsychology, the drive, whose very constitution entails the notion of representation; the Freudian drive is no longer just a drive for discharge. Almost to the contrary, in some sense, the drive comes into being as 'the psychical representative of the stimuli originating from within the organism, and reaching the mind as a measure of the demand made upon the mind for work in consequence of its connection with the body' (Freud, 1915, pp. 121–22).

For Bion, as well, the early accumulation of stimuli is identified as 'the conceptual precursor of the beta phenomena' (Mawson, 2017). As Bion's own thinking developed, however, he moved away from Freud by not following Freud's trajectory from his account of an accumulation of quantity within the mental apparatus to his conception of the drive. Instead, Bion advanced his own metapsychology based on a constellation of concepts (like b-screen and b-elements and *β-phenomena),* all of which are core constructs in Bion's model of dreamwork-alpha (α-function), and belong in his theory of container-contained. Further, it seems to me that Bion's own trajectory, in and of itself, designates the limits of the affinity between Freud's concept of the drive and his own b-elements: while drive remains a representative of the somatic, b-elements are core constructs in Bion's model that pertain to the mind, to the dream-work alpha, encompassed in his 'Theory of Thinking'; the links with the somatic are no longer quite as present.

Freud's 1915 conceptualisation, as already noted, lends itself most significantly to the study of the conjunction of the mental and the somatic. This definition preserves the link between the soma as physiological organism and the mind, and thus the drive serves as a mediating concept which can elucidate the 'leap' between the psychic and the somatic. It acts as a bridge, helping us to understand and work with physically ill patients. As discussed in Section II: 'Clinical pictures', the Freudian concept of the drive in its bridge function, and developed as it is by the Paris School of Psychosomatics, allows for a clinically serviceable understanding of the transformation in patients like Jasmine and Kate, at the time of the development of physical illness.

Furthermore, the bridge concept of the drive helps us move away from an exclusive consideration of either the psychic or the somatic realm. With the concept of the drive, we move away from purely somatic functioning to the domain of the psyche: the domain of internal object representations created psychically by drive cathexis, the domain of narcissism, and the domain of psychic elaboration. In other words, the concept of the drive enabled us to explore the different registers where Jasmine's struggle was coming into existence, shaping the life of the analysis.

This *bridge concept* is precisely the one which from my perspective is lacking in Bion's theory of container/contained, where beta elements belong. Bion's model veers away from the physicality of the soma as such. For him, it seems to me, it is only the body as a conception of the mind that is of relevance to psychoanalysis. The actual physical soma as the source of energy is not an object suitable for psychoanalytic inquiry. Bion, or at least the way his theories have been received and developed, claims that only the workings of the mind can qualify as objects of psychoanalytic exploration (Bronstein, 2015) If that should be the case, one can see that bridging concepts, yoking the psychic and the somatic, would not be of interest – or even pertinent – within Bion's theory.

To conclude, from the perspective outlined above, I have come to think that it is difficult to envisage how the concept of beta elements, notwithstanding their theoretical affinity with the concept of the drive, can be of service either in studying transformations like the one Jasmine went through at the period of somatisation, or in the study of the development of her somatic symptoms. It may be that further study and re-conceptualisation of the mechanisms underlying the a and b phenomena, on the one hand, and of the status of the actual soma in Bion's theory, on the other, could open up new avenues of understanding and working clinically with physically ill patients from the perspective of his metapsychology. But that work remains to be done.

CHRISTIAN SEULIN

In a view that is consistent with the idea of a psychosomatic unity, following Freud, drives appear like forces which, originating in the soma, find expression in the individual's psychic life and behaviour. This is why Freud (1915) claims that the drive is a limit concept on the border of the psychic and the somatic. *Affects* – and we can refer to Freud's notion of 'quota of affect' (Freud, 1915) consist of the drive's energetic manifestation that is qualified at the psychic level. The drives originate in the soma, and their psychic elaboration consists first as the creation of a representative of the drive where there is no distinction between representation and affect, and later as the couple of ideational representative and affect representative. What I call 'qualification of affects' is when the energy (the pure quota) gets linked with differentiated affects (i.e. guilt, shame, joy, pain, sadness etc.), which constitutes the affect representative.

In the treatment, the emergence of affects reflects the dynamics of the drives, and a variety of states may evolve in the course of the work, exclusively or not. With the somatising patients in the clinical cases presented in this book, several states seem to prevail over others: affective suppression, emotional excess with little qualification in terms of affects, as well as the emergence of affects on the side of the analyst in his or her countertransference.

The drive, a necessary hypothesis in psychoanalysis according to Freud, can be seen as what impels the individual; in its most developed form, the drive may find a psychic and then a relational outcome, but it can also be expressed in the body or behaviour, circumventing psychic elaboration. To borrow Francis Pasche's phrase, 'repetition is the instinct of the drive'. At best, repetition can take place in order to elaborate, but the compulsion to repeat reflects the hurdles in the work of psychic elaboration, as it does in dreams in the case of traumatic neurosis.

In 1915, Freud put forward a definition of the drive where it was endowed with certain qualities: constant pressure, a source, an aim, and an object. This definition concurred with Freud's drive theory at the time: his opposition of ego drives and object drives, which followed the opposition of self-preservation drives and sexual drives. The introduction of the death drive in 1920 brought about a new and final opposition: Eros *vs* Thanatos, life drives *vs* death drives. From then on, the 1915 definition of the drive's qualities could no longer be applied.

The 1920 drive-related opposition between life and death drives continues to spark debate, even though no one can deny how considerable a place destructiveness holds in mental as well as somatic pathologies. Should such destructiveness be referred to as the death drive, however? What would a theory of the drives that is congruent with today's biological knowledge be like? From my perspective, cellular apoptosis (Amaisen, 1999) cannot be taken as evidence of the existence of the death drive. It relates to regulation phenomena within a group of cells following an instinctual programme. At an international level, many analysts have jettisoned the concept of drive, but in my view it would be like jettisoning the idea of some energy thrust rooted in the somatic, when the effects of this is frequently revealed to us in everyday clinical observation. In part, such defiance against the drive theory in many analysts probably originates in the quasi-philosophical dimension of Freud's final drive duality. I think that the drive concept is irreplaceable, but I do not agree with Freud's later drive theory, Eros *vs* Thanathos, because I do not think that drive has anything to do with any aim or meaning, even life or death. Drive is only the quality of a being, and the proof and the effect of his psychic development rooted in the soma, in his environment, and in his experiences.

Conflict dwells at the heart of life. And so Freud's general dualist reflections are precious; yet in all of Freud's oppositions we might need to envisage both of his terms as non-homogeneous, i.e. not of the same order. Thus, in my view, and in accordance with Green (Green, 1997), the drive and the object make up two poles of an indivisible duality, but they are in no way of the same order. The representative of the drive (instinctual representative in the *Standard Edition*) combines the ideational representative and the affective representative, two terms that are of a distinct nature as well. Eros's aim in Freud's last drive theory is to bring together ever larger components, whereas Thanatos consists in destroying, unbinding. Should we endorse the theory of a duality of the drives when the binding-unbinding opposition observable in clinical practice is not really explained by the Eros–Thanatos opposition: the opposition of construction and chaos might not necessarily imply the existence of Eros and Thanatos. The Freudian model of the life and death drives relies on a theorisation that arises from Greek philosophy (Empedocles) and on the thermodynamic models of his time.

Physics and physiological phenomena are probably more complex and less clearly in opposition than in Freud's late drive theory. Why not think that, at its source, the sexual drive is formless, objectless, and aimless; it is a mere impetus originating in a somatic source, seeking direction, simply guided in its initial movement by innate biological programmes, which Bion refers to as 'preconceptions'. The study of infantile development has taught us that there exist times in early life that are conducive to the activation of such innate programmes (ref); after these times, the capacities for realisation will no longer be available, sometimes in an irreversible fashion. The somatic drive subsequently discharges and follows pathways that are either anarchic or trace sadomasochistic solutions rooted in trauma, and can find an outlet in compulsive or impulse behaviour, if not in the soma.

While in Freud's 1915 account, the capacities for symbolisation reflect the drive's vectorising psychisation and organise the psyche, what comes later under the death drive seems more complex to me. Under the designation of the death drive, I think we see the failure of the drive's psychic elaboration through different modalities. The death drive gathers failures of various natures: the chaos of the formless drive impetus, i.e. the excitation; the sexualising effects of traumas; the narcissistic negativity stemming from despair tied to failures of satisfactions; the weight of alienating identifications and the destructive perverse models.

If we wish to discuss the cases of Cate and Jasmine from the perspective of drives and affects, we can see the impact of traumas, of repetition compulsion, and of the insufficient psychic elaboration of the drive. But I would like to say a few things about the central place of the countertransference in reflecting the dynamics of drives and affects in the analytic work of these two cases. The countertransference effectively reflects these two patients' expectations regarding the object. In Cate's case, the analyst's countertransference feelings reveal that a defective object, which has not survived, is at stake. In Jasmine's case, the countertransference conveys the mother's inhumane demand of prematurity from the child that the patient once was, which enables the analyst to explore a primary maternal transference and the elaboration of related traumas. The manifestations of the unconscious are therefore featured in the countertransference. Such manifestations consist in drive-related derivatives that direct us regarding the transferential stake. From the point of view of the transference-countertransference theory in the treatment, we could say that any objectifying formulation of the patient's functioning is stamped with the transference-countertransference dynamics in the session. In a nutshell, and referring to what we know now in the scientific field, the observer is a stake in the observed, just as the observed interacts on the basis of what he or she perceives in the observer and his or her position.

I must unfortunately limit myself to only a few aspects of these rich clinical presentations. In the case of Cate, negative countertransference affects arise in the analyst from the outset, which might have been induced by the nature of the patient's phone message as well as by the mix-up regarding the doorbell at the first meeting. This negative induction, which some might refer to as projective identification, should in my view be understood as Cate's quest for the analyst to somehow host her anarchic drive-related dynamics, experienced by Cate as destructive to the object. From the start, Cate reveals that she strives to find an object that might accept her and bear her violence by surviving and without retaliating. The patient displays strong emotions with tears, which show she has difficulty qualifying affects, in a clinical picture that calls to mind actual neurosis with automatic anxiety. The anxiety is tied to the constant anticipation of abandonment, and the traumas pertain to her relational failures, the first one involving a mother who did not love her or give her anything. The corollary of this meaningless emotional discharge (the patient says that her life is devoid of meaning, that she is behaving like a child) is the difficulty she encounters developing phantasmatic activity. We see the analyst carrying out this work of phantasmisation on her behalf and developing affectivity within himself, which somehow compensates for the deficiency in his patient.

Cate's difficulty resurfaces in the dream in which she is looking at paintings in an art gallery and suddenly they disappear: obliteration of representations, blanking of thought. The breast cancer traumatism, the impact of her treatments, and the shadow cast by a worrisome prognosis, could perhaps be held responsible for such representational bewilderment. Was there a psychological element predisposing this impulsive and immature woman to cancer, she who mainly relied on behavioural strategies? Indeed, in Cate's case, defiant behaviour at school and the resort to sexuality and alcohol are long-standing strategies that reflect a search for drive-related discharge rather than elaboration. Another feature of her character has seemed to damage her capacities for drive elaboration: in the face of frustration, and in particular in response to the pain inherent in the link with the mother (further enhanced by the mother's assumed preference for her brother), she has been defending herself via evacuation, rejection, and a form of pseudo-indifference based on a negative narcissistic carapace. Only with the threat of cancer and undertaking therapy may suffering and depression resurface. While previously she disclosed nothing to others of her emotional states, she was in fact 'fuming' internally. The preconscious pathways of drive transformation could be said to have been obstructed, between a cold cognitive pole defended narcissistically and an unconscious furnace full of undifferentiated excitation.

The case of Jasmine raises other questions from the perspective of drive-related dynamics. Jasmine comes to see the analyst expressing a 'wish for analysis' because of a feeling of futility in her life where 'all is grey'. She explains that she is in an excellent professional and social situation, a good marriage, with two daughters who fulfil her. She is the youngest of four, has always experienced herself as the 'apple of her father's eyes', which made the other children envious, especially her sisters. According to what she says about her childhood, she had a happy family. The analyst notices the urgency she conveys through her behaviour when she arrives and when the meeting comes to an end. She also wonders about the motives underlying her wish for analysis, motives which leave her perplexed despite brief moments when some pain and turmoil seemingly come through. The impression drawn from this initial meeting is that, at bottom, Jasmine does everything she can to present an idyllic picture of her life in a composed, rational and defensive way, suppressing all the affects connoting pain, violence or depression. Her verbal expression is rather smooth, polished and delicate, keeping the analyst as well as herself at a distance from her affects, like a description from without that hides a lived experience she keeps quiet about. Emotions show through, however, in the urgency at both ends of the session and a few gaps in her speech signalling pain and turmoil. We could say that the feeling of futility that Jasmine complains about mirrors her speech, which lacks the ballast of affects and has evacuated the density of imagoes. All that remains is the non-conflictual image of a worshipped father. As soon as the analyst attempts to suggest the possibility of conflict among the siblings during the first meeting, or questions the preventive motives of her demand for analysis in the second meeting, the patient skilfully evades the offer to acknowledge conflict. The analyst identifies a need to run away from any emotional contact with her, even by 'forgetting' the analyst's presence (is this the effect of her denial, or her erasure of the analyst?). Feeling emotions would make her appear vulnerable.

Yet, Jasmine does not seem to function on an operative mode, as basic affects only become visible in her occasionally; in this case too, the countertransference signals conflicts inside the patient who does not seem to feel the conflict: the analyst recurrently experiences the feeling of an 'unmotivated' demand for analysis, as if her patient could manage by herself, which the analyst subtly ties to the patient's object history and to an identification. The rest of the treatment will show the unfurling of a negative maternal transference in relation to a cold mother with low affect who could have been dangerous for her children. The traumatic dimension of the link to this mother will be experienced in the transference, and it elicits the elaborative examination of this transference via homosexual dynamics restorative of the maternal deficiency – the primary one mainly, but also the secondary one (the sexed female body). Once again, it is up to the analyst, identified with the patient's mother, to experience in her countertransference the affect of disgust at the breastfeeding baby, leading to a possible interpretation of the trauma.

In the treatment, the emergence of hypochondria and of somatic symptoms (tinnitus, breast cysts) along with invasive anxiety, indeed coincides with the return of the trauma and of the affects of hate, as well as of the quest for a maternal relationship. They at once convey the search for a link with the object as close as possible to the body, and reflect the economic overload tied to the return of the traumatism that was until then kept at a distance probably through splitting. The lifting of such a split exposes the patient to a drive-related outburst that affects both soma and psyche. And among the various symptoms she presents in this climate of automatic anxiety, some are clearly functional and symbolic – such as tachycardia tied to frustrated erotic impulses, if not tinnitus – and others are of a proven organic somatic nature, such as the breast cysts.

As regards the two cases discussed in the present context, emphasis must be laid on the difficulties relating to the Oedipal organisation as well as to the organisation of the primal fantasies. These treatments are primarily centred on the link with the maternal object. Whether we are dealing with the anarchy of drive-related behavioural solutions, as in Cate's case, or with the ideal organisation of relational and social life to counter drives and conflicts, as in Jasmine's case, the structuring of the oedipus complex seems to be difficult and not really functioning. The same can be said about the primal scene fantasy which organises psychic life. Indeed, through their development and their effectiveness, the oedipus complex and the primal fantasies reflect the degree of drive elaboration, endowing the drive with flexible psychic forms likely to represent desire in its active and passive variants with qualified affects. In the cases discussed, the obstruction of the work of symbolisation seems to affect the very organisation of the hallucinatory satisfaction of desire, especially in Cate's case.

Commentary

JÖRG FROMMER

In her contribution, Marina Perris highlights what could be called the paradox of the drive concept. The drive is a core metapsychological concept of psychoanalysis, which represents the economic aspects of psychic life. But the definition of the drive varies throughout Freud's works. The variation of definitions of this limit concept between the psyche and soma increases dramatically if we take into account not only the work of Freud but other prominent psychoanalytic authors.

Marina exemplifies this in her analysis, comparing Freud's definition of drive with Bion's concept of beta elements; what appear to be very similar at first sight crystallise as rather different under the microscope of Marina's critical investigation. Whereas Freud came from a background in biology and always kept the soma in mind throughout his life, Bion's theoretical thinking, Marina writes, 'veers away' from the body as a biological fact that has an economic impact on psychic life, and only takes into account the psychic representation of the body. Comparing the different definitions of the beta element concept through the writings of Bion, Marina shows that the definitions vary significantly. In another main difference between Freud and Bion, Marina argues that in Bion beta elements stay untransformed without the activity of the alpha-function, but in Freud the drive concept itself encompasses transformation activities from the physical towards the mental. In her discussion, Marina criticises Bion's dualistic exclusion of the biological sphere from his theory of mental processes and calls for an integrative view, allowing for a better understanding of somatic symptoms from the perspective of metapsychology.

Christian Seulin's remarks are in concordance with Marina's statement in so far as he also accepts the drive concept as a basic model for psychoanalytic psychosomatics. However, Christian's use of the concept of drive comes with doubts. He warns of an uncritical use of the death drive concept for chaotic and destructive processes in general, keeping in mind that the regulation of physiological processes is usually complex and can rarely be explained unilaterally by a single cause. This implies, regarding the clinical case of Cate, that the breast cancer she came down with should not be prematurely misinterpreted as caused by (death) drive forces, because too many questions regarding the interaction of somatic disease and psychic decompensation are unclear and unanswered. Nevertheless, under Christian's perspective both clinical cases demonstrate psychic vulnerability due to traumatisation, which arises in part from the primary caretaking by the mother in early childhood.

In Marina's interpretation, the somatic symptoms that appear in the sixth year of analysis of Jasmine are an expression of 'drive activity mobilised by intense erotic feelings in the transference' based on early traumatic experiences in her life history. According to Christian's remarks, Jasmine's somatisation results in specific countertransference configurations that reflect different degrees of drive elaboration; whereas in Cate, the traumatic experience of a 'defective object that has not survived' results in the difficulty of organising phantasmatic activity at all, and forces the analyst to carry out compensating mentalisation on her behalf, in Jasmine phantasmatic activity is preserved, but the 'relation to a cold mother' results in negative countertransference feelings.

Why is the decision to use or not use the drive concept in interpretations of clinical case work important? In my view, the main problem of the drive concept is that it implies a denial of the unbridgeable methodological dualism between a hermeneutic access to the patient using *understanding* in communication as the essential medium of analytic work, and a natural science access using *measuring* of physiological dysfunctions and structural organ damages. Instead of using a 'bridge concept' for phenomena from different realms of methodologically incompatible world experiences, I would rather propose that we avoid bridging the unbridgeable. This leads to an acceptance of the gap between our understanding of psychic phenomena and their somatic roots. The consequence for clinical interpretations is that we are aware of the fact that the more we introduce somatic factors as relevant to our metapsychological understanding, the more the uncertainty of the truth claim of these interpretations increases.

Maybe even Freud was aware of these basic problems of theorisation of drive activity when he – as Christian quotes–wrote about 'quota of affect' and thus differentiated between two aspects intermingled in the drive concept: on the one hand, the psychological aspect of *affect*, accessible solely by the extraction of the rules of inner experience via subtle qualitative phenomenological content description; and on the other hand, the aspect of *quota*, following economic laws, accessible mainly by the measurement of physiological parameters. Taking seriously as well the 'affect' as the 'quota' aspect, I would like to propose, as I have pointed out in Chapter 9 of this book, that we respect the methodological dualism, and we introduce the primitive aspects of psychic life into metapsychology by widening the field of semantics to semiotics, rather than jumping over fragile bridges from psychology into biology.

Regarding our need for theorisation, from a psychoanalytical point of view we should keep in mind that theories are always incomplete attempts at reducing the complexity of the experienced world. Thus, sometimes this process of theorisation will primarily serve the reduction of the analyst's difficulties of bearing the complexity which he or she has not always fully understood. In line with this argument, Jacques Press (2016) recently proposed a theoretical thinking open to ambiguity, formlessness, and the negative. In my opinion, the drive is an obsolete and antiquated concept if we understand it in its concrete, naturalistic meaning, but it is a fruitful heuristic concept if we understand it in its tentativeness.

Note

1 As I understand it, Freud postulates that the stimuli originate from within the organism. A process is then initiated and through its unfolding a demand for work is eventually placed upon the mind. It is in the meeting of this demand that the drive is constituted as the psychic representative of the somatic.

References

Aisenstein, M. (2006) 'The indissociable unity of psyche and soma: a view from the Paris Psychosomatic School', *Int. J. Psychoanal.*, 87, pp. 667–80.

Aisenstein, M. (2010) 'The Mysterious Leap of the Somatic into the Psyche' in *Psychosomatics Today: A Psychoanalytic Perspective*. London: Karnac.

Amaisen, J.C. (1999) *La sculpture du vivant*. Paris: Le Seuil.

Bion, W.F. (1962) *Learning from Experience*. London: Tavistock.

Bion, W.F (1962) 'A Theory of Thinking', *Int. J. Psychoanal.*, 43, 4–5.

Bion, W.F. (1963) *Elements of Psychoanalysis* London: Heinemann.

Bion, W.F. (1967) *Second Thoughts*. London: Heinemann.

Bion, W.F. (1992) *Cogitations*. London: Karnac.

Freud, S. and Breuer, J. (1955[1895d]) 'Studies on hysteria', *S.E., Vol. 2*. London: The Hogarth Press.

Bronstein, C. (2015) 'Contributions from British Psychoanalysts', British-German Colloquium conference, Heidelberg.

Freud, S. (1900). *The Interpretation of Dreams. S.E., Vol. 2*. London: The Hogarth Press.

Freud, S. (1905) 'Three Essays on Sexuality', *S.E., Vol. 7*. London: The Hogarth Press.

Freud, S. (1915) 'Instincts and their Vicissitudes', *S.E., Vol. 14*. London: The Hogarth Press.

Green, A. (1997) *Les chaînes d'Eros*. Paris: Odile Jacob.

Green, A. (1998) 'The primordial mind and the work of the negative', *Int. J. Psychoanal.*, 79, 649–64.

Green, A. (2005) *Psychoanalysis: A Paradigm for Clinical Thinking*. London: Free Association Books.

Kohon, G. (2014) 'Making contact with the primitive mind: The contact-barrier, beta-elements and the drive', *Int. J. Psychoanal.*, 95, 245–70.

Marty, P. (1958) 'La relation objectale allergique', *Revue française de psychanalyse*, 22, 1, pp. 7–30.

Marty, P. (1968) 'A Major Process of Somatization: The Progressive Disorganization', *Int. J. Psychoanal.*, 49, pp. 246–49.

Mawson, C. (2017) 'Notes on "postscript on beta elements"', in Working with somatic patients: The concept of the drive". *Bulletin of the British Psychoanalytic society*, 53(2), February 2017.

Perris, M. (2014) 'Working with psychosomatic patients: the concept of the drive', *Revue française de psychosomatique*, 48.

Press, J. (2016) 'Metapsychological and clinical issues in psychosomatics research', *Int. J. Psychoanal.*, 97, pp. 89–113.

Reed, G.S., Levine, H.B. and Scarfone, B. (2013) 'Introduction: From a universe of presences to a universe of absences', in Reed, G.S., Levine, H.B. and Scarfone, B. (eds), *Unrepresented States and the Construction of Meaning: Clinical and Theoretical Contributions*. London: Karnac.

Smadja, C. (2005) *The Psychosomatic Paradox*. London: Free Association Books.

Smajda, C. (2011) 'Psychoanalytic psychosomatics', *Int. J. Psychoanal.*, 92, pp. 221–30.

Chapter 7

Ideal ego, ego ideal and superego

BÉRENGÈRE DE SENARCLENS

In this chapter, we will consider how agencies such as the ideal ego, the ego ideal and superego might relate to the somatisation process. To start, I would like to try to give clearer definitions of these notions before I turn to how I think they operate in the clinical material. Let us begin with the 'ideal ego' since it is the most archaic agency and coincides with quite an unorganised ego. Freud theorises the ideal ego (Freud, 1914) in order to designate the primitive ego tied to the narcissistic ideal, which is marked by infantile omnipotence. The ideal ego is an unconscious narcissistic phenomenon, unrelated to later identifications with love objects. It develops in an early stage that corresponds to an ideal condition before the child encounters the actual frustrations of his needs in relation to reality. Somehow, throughout their lives, human beings desperately try, at an unconscious level, to re-experience this narcissistic fusional ideal and its omnipotence.

We could say that the ideal ego is a *limited* intrapsychic formation. In this primitive period of life, preconscious and developed representations are poor. Megalomania and a need for perfection originate in this phase of primary narcissism. At this stage, the ideal ego is not negotiable: it appears as an imperative in order to survive, not just a wish but a question of life or death. The demands of the ideal ego of narcissistic omnipotence are tyrannical, persecutory and without limits. They are defined by excessiveness and by an inexhaustible demand on oneself and others. Sometimes the ideal ego develops in the form of heroic fantasies in which the child sees himself accomplishing thousands of wonders. The voracity of the subject is such that he *wants all, all at the same time and right away*. This logic, which we might call a *primary logic*, certainly does not take reality into account. Similarly, if the ideal ego is impinged upon, it is experienced as shame or annihilation in a very binary way. The ideal ego is the heir to a fantasy of fusion with the object. Originating early in life, it is always related to the body but essentially to the maternal object which is seen as ideal too.

Let us continue with definitions and differentiate between the ideal ego, as described above, and the superego and ego ideal structures which are *intrapsychic* and result from secondary identifications. The ego ideal, as defined by Freud in 1923, is part of the superego, heir to the oedipus complex. This structure has a kind of protective function and reflects a better integrated and more solid ego. The ego ideal, linked with the identification process, contains the future object choices and represents *the one I would like to be*. It refers to the positive values which the subject strives towards. The ego ideal is linked *in fine* to the satisfaction felt when faced with representations invested as good and positive, and it implies a sufficiently good integration of reality. The ego ideal is related to the way in which the subject has to behave in order to satisfy the authority's demand. In that respect, the superego reproduces the authority of the parent-child relationship; it is a critical internal agency very much linked to the fear of losing the love and security of the objects.

As we can see, ideal ego and superego/ego ideal structures are two different forms of *inheritance*; they refer to two periods of ego development: pre- and post-oedipal. Under the influence of the limitations of reality, the ego development is a long process – it takes place through the integration of the drives and through object relations, which allow for a transformation, at least partial, of the archaic ideal ego into a well-integrated superego and ego ideal structure; it is a long process until superego and ego ideal become 'trustful inhabitants of the ego' as Antonino Ferro has put it (Ferro, 2010). This development is not without obstacles and complications.

In other words, if the superego/ego ideal is a 'sufficiently solid' structure, and if the quality of the 'subjective appropriation' (Roussillon, 2007, pp. 3–9) is good too, this results in adequate defence mechanisms and a healthy psychic development. But if the superego/ego ideal is not sufficiently strong, then the primitive ideal ego, with its magical thinking, takes the lead, weakening the superego. Under psychically stressful circumstances, an apparently well-integrated oedipal superego might not prevent the strong reactivation of an archaic ideal ego in its sadistic and absolute manner, following its particular primary logic, its primitive narcissistic defences, along with shame or primary guilt, which often come with the primary conviction that the subject is responsible for the destruction of the object.

We observe that in this type of regression it sometimes looks as if the ideal ego, and its logic of omnipotence, were *used* paradoxically as a kind of magical tool to control things and prevent the return of the distress linked to a primary traumatic state. This distinctly illusive defence seems to be tied to a sudden or more general deficiency in mentalisation and to an inability to metabolise drives. Let us now insist on the role of traumatic experiences in this context. Trauma is what overwhelms the psyche. It is an excitement that cannot be contained, either by a too fragile ego or by the primary objects. The primary trauma invades the subject and becomes persecutory. It really seems that the ideal ego is somehow contemporary with old primitive traumatic experiences. In this context of *too much* for the child's ability, we can observe how ejection and splitting become unavoidable defence mechanisms in a desperate attempt to preserve the ideals of fusion and omnipotence.

The mechanism of splitting is a real amputation. The evacuation it entails seems to emerge as a vital necessity for the primitive self. The more precocious the splitting, the more disabling it will be. It requires a lot of energy from the patient because it is as if he needed to maintain control over that split, over what it contains, and at the same time, paradoxically, as if he had to deal with contradictory forces – the compulsion to repeat and the compulsion to represent. Such 'forces' strive to disclose what is contained in the split, since it is also clearly full of true and vital elements. The splitting mechanism is undoubtedly more related to the ideal ego than to the superego structure.

One answer to a traumatic invasion and the 'loss' it generated (through splitting or ejection) could be somatisation; it is as if no real capacity for symbolisation or representation would 'stop' that process. Therefore, traumatic experiences could become a fertile ground for the development of psychosomatic disorganisations. Perhaps, later on in life, the prospect of a loss might awaken the violence of some ideal ego logic with its narcissistic omnipotence. In other words, any feeling of grief could pave the way for the re-emergence of earlier unsymbolised losses, bringing about regression and temporal confusion. Sometimes patients come to analysis with the mad unconscious secret that the treatment will magically repair that loss and confusion.

I agree with Jacques Press that some of these early experiences are 'unforgettable' in the sense that the primitive unrepresented traces, which haunt the psyche, remain unintegrated. The subject constantly ejects them, but the traumatic experiences remain as they are, without any modification over time. It is in this way that they are unforgettable. These unrepresented traumatic elements struggle to be expressed in words; sometimes verbal expression fails and so they express themselves via the body or enactments. We could argue that the more something is denied, split or unknown, the more it might solicit a somatic form of expression. As analysts, we are called upon to try to grasp this type of language and transform it into words. In this context, I think I need to clarify the term ego. When I use this term, I am not referring to the id-ego-superego triad of the second topography, but rather to the ego as a container as well as the contained. In fact, the ego as the result of the whole process of *subjective appropriation* and the development of the mentalisation–symbolisation processes.

In its construction, the ego will progressively 'part' from a 'non-ego'; the subject will part from the primal object and this will allow for, in time, the integration of a 'third'. This ego non-ego differentiation is a much earlier process than the differentiation of sexes or generations. It is constructed concurrently with the capacity to say 'no', which is at the basis of identity. In my view, such a 'construction', which relates to infantile drive activity as well as to the reaction of the environment, implies the inseparability of drive theory and object relations theory.

In other words, clinically speaking, when the object seemingly did not play the role of container and mediator during early childhood, the ideal ego usually takes hold of the psyche with its potentially destructive consequences. The patient clings to this omnipotence and, I would say, to a kind of primary logic. This strange and illusionary defence takes up the whole space, leaving no room for a more secondary logic or differentiated post-oedipal structure. There is a difficulty in dealing with drives in general because they cannot be metabolised.

It seems that too much ideal ego, along with the deficient development of a solid ego superego structure, a poor introjection of a containing capacity, and finally inadequate symbolisation processes, could be a kind of open door to somatisation. To state this differently, let us ask: could a fragmented, badly integrated ego be one of the factors leading to somatisation? Could it be equivalent to a fragile immune system, which cannot offer sufficient defences against somatic illnesses? Would a fortified ego, a sufficiently good psychic economy, enriched with a solid superego and ego ideal structure, provide some kind of protection against certain forms of somatisation?

Cate and Jasmine

I would now like to link these thoughts with the clinical material presented in the book. It seems to me that the two cases somehow illustrate some of what I have expressed above. These two patients are different in many respects, but in both cases we can observe from the beginning an unrepresented conflict between contradictory feelings. The decision to consult an analyst might signal traces of magic infantile idealisation and expectation, a desperate hope to find a psychic place yet to be found. These two patients confront us right away with a paradox: an illusion and an expected disillusion. This seems tied to elements of what we could call an *ideal ego climate*. With these two patients, strong unconscious positive and negative transferences are felt from the outset, along with the scars of primary traumatic states. There is a climate of *too much* in the air.

In both cases, the ego seems fragile, with many split parts. The ego and non-ego separation is not clear. The defence against such a state seemingly consists in holding on to and ideal ego, full of omnipotence but also harsh demands. Therefore, both patients seem to live in a kind of survival mode. The full *appropriation* of the various elements of their experiences and affects seems hazardous and daunting. Ejection is therefore the privileged defence mechanism.

Technically one has the impression that both analysts, each in their own way, are striving to recognise and verbalise on behalf of their patients the two movements of the conflict; they attempt to verbalise what looks like a split, and they try to uncover what seems to be negative transference, with the hate and wrath that come with it. This is a lengthy process. Sometimes the two levels – pre and post-oedipal – are involved and it seems that both require an interpretation. At some point, Fotis chooses to interpret the body movement as a kind of masturbation; it appears clear that this material is also an expression of something more primitive, that we can link maybe with the notion of hospitalism used by René Spitz. The difficulty in these cases is that the two levels of organisation are constantly present.

But, as the treatment progresses, both patients come out of what looked like a subject-object confusion. In both cases, the ideal ego turns towards a more realistic ego ideal. Little by little, the borders of the ego allow for a better containing capacity, for less anxiety about being invaded or abandoned, and more stability. In other words, it seems that the drives, the beta elements, are more integrated. There is less fear of imminent disaster in connection with a *too much.* The integration of an object *in absentia* is more stable. Are the superego and the ego ideal becoming trustful and helpful? To conclude, I would say that for these two patients the somatic attack somehow seems to have provided an opportunity, an open door to the verbal expression of affects which were formerly unrepresentable.

NICK TEMPLE

In considering the role of the ideal ego, ego ideal, and the superego in psychosomatic conditions, we need to understand how these concepts are defined at the present time and the contribution they make to understanding the origin of psychosomatic states.

As Britton (Britton, 2003, p. 104) points out, it is often said that there has been a confusing interchange of terms since Freud introduced the term ego ideal. The question has been raised as to whether it is the same as ideal ego. And is it the same as the superego? Freud at times used ego ideal and superego interchangeably. When he used only one or other term interchangeably in this way, he attributed two functions to the agency: to act as an ideal model, and to act as the critical agency that judged how the individual measured up to this ideal. By 1923, the superego had become well-established in Freud's thinking as the internalisation of parental authority: 'of these two identifications (father and mother) in some way united with each other as an ego ideal or superego' (Freud, 1923b). Freud brings forward the view that the critical function of the superego constitutes an agency which has become separate from the ego and that dominates it, as is shown by pathological states of mourning or melancholia where the subject feels he is the brunt of criticism and denigration: 'We see how one part of the ego sets itself over and against the other, judges it critically and as it were takes it as its object' (Freud, 1923b).

By 1930, the concept of the superego was established as the seat of conscience and its punitive nature was emphasised. Freud (1930a, p. 130) attributed the aggression of the superego to the projection of aggression of a young child onto its parental precursors, acknowledging this to be the suggestion of Melanie Klein. At this point, the nomenclature seems to become clearer. Freud says that 'the perfection which the child attributed to them (the parents) now acquires a new meaning' (Freud, 1930a). If we take it that the child has already attributed an existing phantasy of an ideal-self to the parents, he then introjects the model self-ideal and parental-ideal as one and the same. As Britton (2003, p. 106) points out, the religious version of this dynamic would be Christ's words, 'Believe me that I am in the Father and the Father is in me'. Freud added to this theological understanding with the suggestion that the child's superego is modelled not on the parent, but on the parent's superego: 'You should not simply listen to me' the parent might say, 'but listen to the father inside me' (Freud, 1933a).

Britton's (2003, pp. 107–12) discussion of the book of Job in relation to the superego and ego is relevant to this discussion and to the consideration of somatisation as arising at the point of conflict between the superego and the ego. Job is afflicted with loathsome sores and illness by God. In this conflict, Job becomes capable of complaining about God as unrelenting and incapable of change, a great failing if he were to be judged as a man. This is perhaps another example of the idea of emancipation from the superego, where the ego can challenge the cruel aspects of the superego. This resembles the change that can occur in analysis when the patient acquires the capacity to challenge the harsh judgement of the superego, for example in recovering from a severe depression. It raises the question of whether it is important to consider this movement when a patient shifts from being afflicted by somatic symptoms to being able to symbolise the ambivalent conflict with the superego figure – both in dreams and in the exploration of the transference relationship with the analyst. The analyst's countertransference is an important way of understanding this situation. For example, when Marina Perris's patient Jasmine experiences her analyst as rejecting, in the initial countertransference the analyst finds she is puzzled as to why the patient needs an analysis. But in the second consultation the analyst does come to understand the patient's distress and need for help.

In psychosomatic illness there is clinical evidence to suggest the possibility that psychosomatic symptoms can provide a way of containing a persecutory internal relationship with a critical superego figure, which becomes located in the patient's body through a process of displacement and somatisation. The psychic conflict is transformed into a physical symptom in which the body is subject to the painful conflict. This is dramatically illustrated in auto-immune conditions where the body's immune defences are turned against itself. This occurs for example in eczema and asthma.

Aisenstein's (2006) concept of acting in the body is important in this situation. With Marina's patient Jasmine, there is an enactment with a symbolic function displaced into the body resulting in a somatic symptom. This can be linked to other forms of acting out where a phantasy is enacted, sometimes directly related to the transference. The problem of acting in the body is more difficult to conceptualise and to understand in view of the neural and hormonal pathways that may be involved. Damasio's (1994) work emphasises how much the mind and body function as one entity, echoing Freud's view that the ego is always a body-ego.

The anxiety and suffering of symptoms may represent the guilt which the patient experiences in relation to conflict in the internal relationship with the superego. This was evident in the famous case of Charles Darwin. He was able to think and to formulate his concepts, but he was fearful of publishing them. While working on his great theory of evolution he suffered from tormenting psychosomatic symptoms and fearful hypochondriasis. It was as if he was being cruelly punished by his symptoms for his bold and original thinking which challenged orthodox views. This could be compared with the way he consciously feared he would be punished by the church and academic authorities for his creative thinking if he published his theories. This led to twenty years delay in publishing *The Origin of Species*. His evolutionary hypothesis was, of course, controversial and shattering to religious orthodoxy of the time.

One problem in these situations is that the conflict is not able to be represented symbolically, although there is the question of whether the somatic symptom itself partly has a symbolic function, in Segal's terms it might be a symbolic equation, a primitive form of symbolisation (Segal, 1957). This remains a controversial area in psychosomatics. In some instances, when a patient begins to represent the conflict with the superego in dreams and is able to explore the conflict in the transference relationship, there is an improvement in the somatic symptoms. This is more strongly the case if the patient is able to express anger and ambivalence towards the analyst in the transference, which can alleviate the physical symptoms; the persecutory relationship becomes contained by the analyst's understanding of the transference situation and their capacity to respond in a thoughtful way, representing a benign superego that does not repeat or enact a persecutory figure.

Marina's patient Jasmine first puzzled the analyst in the initial consultation; the analyst questioned why she needed help when everything seemed to be going well for her. But following the second consultation in which the analyst was more in touch with the patient's distress, she agreed to take the patient on for analysis. Immediately before the analysis commenced, the patient developed severe abdominal pain, a warning of the later developments of somatic symptoms that would occur – tinnitus, tachycardia and hypertension. From this we can see a vivid picture of a conflicted struggle with a much-desired but rejecting internal figure, represented in the transference relationship. Further symptoms occurred when Jasmine developed cysts in her breast. The dream reported in the later sessions reveals the underlying painful situation in which Jasmine displays herself seductively to Mr K, for whom she has erotic feelings, but he is asleep and does not respond to her. This is followed by her association to the dream in which at the age eleven she remembers displaying herself sexually to her male cousin who humiliatingly rejects her. The dream and the associations can be seen to represent the erotic transference with a humiliating rejection by the much-desired analyst/mother.

It seems that this case illustrates the way in which the patient at certain times in the analysis can only express her vulnerability through the process of somatisation or acting in the body. The patient later remembers her colds and tummy aches as a child, which expressed her distress. She believed her mother was not able to stand her distressed feelings. The patient described having a daydream as a child about a road accident in which she is killed, and she pictured her mother's terrible distress at learning of her death. She thought of this as her retaliatory punishment towards her mother for her indifference to her feelings.

Marina sensitively describes something emerging in the treatment, which she feels obscurely in the countertransference but it remains inaccessible until the development of the further episodes of somatisation, tinnitus, hypertension and tachycardia. Eventually, the somatic progression developed into a dangerous issue of recurrent cysts in her breast. The later stages of the analysis which are reported allowed an exploration of the way in which the somatic symptoms represent the difficult ambivalent relationship with the mother. There is also the exploration of sexualised fantasies about the doctor/analyst examining the patient's breast. Does this represent the erotic transference to the much-desired maternal figure who is painfully rejecting? Or is this a defensive sexualisation of the difficult persecuted relationship with the mother which has become concretely expressed in the somatic symptoms.

We can ask the important question: what are the origins of a persecutory superego which may be contained in psychosomatic states? Do these origins lie in an experience of trauma with a lack of containment by the mother, or are they the result of being projected into by a parent? It is likely that all of these factors play a part in the development of the persecutory situation. In the case of Jasmine, she experienced her mother as not wanting her and rejecting her in her childhood.

Fotis Bobos's patient Cate describes a history of feeling projected into by her mother, and experiences the analyst as trying to shut her out, even before she has met him. Indeed, her analyst's countertransference leads him to feel that he might not want to see her or take her into treatment. He wonders if his failure to hear the doorbell on her first visit had been related to this countertransference or whether the patient enacted her transference by failing to ring the doorbell loudly enough. Either way, a powerful phantasy exists in the patient's mind of a rejecting figure who wishes to keep her out in a hostile way. She also feels that the breast cancer is a punishment for her negative feelings towards her mother. Fotis takes this up directly, leading the patient to describe her feeling of being punished for causing damage to her mother.

The discussion about the patients' feelings about her mother leads to the idea that the patient's mental crossing out of her mother led to her mother's retaliation, where Cate is crossed out and shut out, but is also punished by the cancer. It is important that Cate can explore this with her analyst and feel sad, connecting this with her strong feelings for her father. In this situation, the analyst seems to have become a more containing figure, like her father, a benign superego figure, in the context of her being persecuted and blamed by a harsh superego version of her mother. It is important in this context that Cate is worried about using the tissues and making a mess and spoiling the relationship with her containing analyst.

Later sessions allow Cate to explore fears of the analyst shutting her out and rejecting her, and she develops a capacity to explore this within certain limits. It is interesting that in the last session reported, where Cate is concerned about her negative thoughts, and the analyst raises the idea that she fears him having a negative attitude towards her, she then reports a dream in which a guardian angel is caressing her hair. It might be argued that here sexualisation is a way of dealing with the dangers of the negative transference. There is evidence, however, that the negative thoughts can be explored in the analytic relationship and contained in a way that assists the patient. The question remains as to whether this will lead to a reduction in the somatisation presented by the breast cancer.

Commentary

FOTIS BOBOS

Bérengère de Senarclens and Nick Temple seem to completely agree about the clinical significance of the agencies of the ideal ego, superego, and ego ideal in understanding how psychosomatic symptoms form an expression of acting in the body. However, their approach diverges on theoretical levels, since they come from different schools of thought. The authors usefully attempt to define the concepts of the ideals and the superego, because their definitions in Freud's writings remain somewhat unclear, as he uses the terms interchangeably, starting with ideal ego and ego ideal (Freud, 1914), and continuing with superego-ego ideal, which he clarifies as the internalisation of parental authority, or the parental superego (Freud, 1923b).

Bérengère finds the concept of ideal ego particularly useful. She considers the necessity for a clear distinction between the two concepts: the ideal ego, referred to as a very early 'limited' intrapsychic formation, and the superego or ego ideal, referred to as a post-oedipal intrapsychic agency; they have two quite different heritages, coming from two different periods of life. Bérengère suggests that the reactivation of early traumas defensively brings back into action the ideal ego of narcissistic omnipotence – related to the subject's body, and to the maternal body – which contributes to preserving significant deficits in the representational capacities of the unorganised ego. I would like to suggest that these deficits in the non-differentiation between ego and non-ego could include essential elements of the oral phase and demonstrate a developmental failure to manage anal phase challenges successfully. Nick prefers to use the concept of the cruel superego instead of the ideal ego. He distinguishes this primitive superego from the benign one. In my opinion, even though there is a difference in terminology here, the primitive superego like the ideal ego refers to primitive levels of the ego development.

I think that the two authors agree that these psychic formations are closely connected with primitive anxieties and the struggle for existence in which the subject feels persecuted, or invaded, or the recipient of parental projections, or abandoned by a parental figure. The origins of these formations are to be found in traumatic experiences during the early childhood period. The convergence between Bérengère and Nick becomes more evident in their discussions of the two clinical cases. Both authors emphasise the presence of massive transference enactment by intense countertransferential reactions from the beginning of the analytic encounters. They agree that the patients' progress of psychic elaboration and integration is the result of the analytic work – the well-timed verbalisations of archaic mechanisms such as splitting and projection aimed at the analyst. In particular, the patients' capacity for expressing negative feelings such as hostility and anger towards the analyst, which can be contained in the analytic relationship without fear of retaliation, is of considerable value. Elaboration of the countertransference helps to create a solid ground for the analytic work.

With regard to my thoughts that Cate's back and forth movement was an element equal to masturbation, I mean that Cate uses her whole moving body in an autoerotic way as an erect narcissistic phallus, rather than as an autoerotism located in a genital bodily zone belonging to the genital phase. Conforming to archaic ideals, the phallic narcissism expresses the denial of any lack and opposes passivity by the hypercathexis of activity (Fain, 1991). It seems to me that the main difference in the two authors' theoretical approaches could be based on the controversial hypothesis about the symbolic function of the psychosomatic symptom – the pre-existence or not of an unconscious powerful phantasy that is already an organised psychic conflict.

Nick raises the question of whether 'the somatic symptom itself partly has a symbolic function . . . it might be . . . a primitive form of symbolisation'. Moreover, discussing Jasmine's case, he suggests the idea of 'an enactment with a symbolic function displaced into the body resulting in a somatic symptom'. I think that in this occasion, Nick explores the somatic symptom somehow as analogous to the hysterical one. At another point, he puts forward the interesting idea of 'the somatic symptom representing the emotional pain which isn't expressed in words or feelings'. It seems to me that here he is in accordance with Freud's statement that the patient chooses to be ill instead of guilty. Bérengère suggests that because of the unrepresented traces of traumatic experiences, the subject deals with severe obstacles in his capacity of transforming and integrating them into his intrapsychic world. The somatic symptom is seen as a possible primitive reaction to the traumatic invasion of the primary object, rather than an expression of a psychic conflict. In some cases, the somatic symptom or the acting out could be the only way for the unrepresented traumatic elements to be expressed.

In conclusion, I suppose that Nick is more in favour of the position that the somatic symptom symbolises, although in a primitive form, pre-existing unconscious psychic conflicts. In contrast, Bérengère claims that the traumatic experiences cannot give rise to a representation of the conflict and therefore the somatic symptom has no symbolic function. The possibility of working through these issues with the new object – the analyst – might help the subject to construct meaning through the process of symbolisation. In my opinion, this theoretical controversy might have clinical implications with regard to technique, namely the analyst's attitude towards formulating constructions that are able to open pathways of different meanings and the decision to reinforce mentalisation processes rather than offer interpretations.

References

Aisenstein, M. (2006) 'The indissociable unity of psyche and soma: a view from the Paris Psychosomatic School', *Int. J. Psychoanal.*, 87, pp. 667–80.
Britton, R. (2003) *Sex, Death and the Superego*. London: Karnac.
Damasio, A. (1994) *Descartes' Error, Emotion, Reason, and the Human Brain*. New York: G.P. Putnam's Sons.
Fain, M. (1991) 'Préambule à une métapsychologie de la vie opératoire', *Revue française de psychosomatique*, 1, pp. 59–79.
Ferro, A. (2010) Paper given at the CPRS Conference, Geneva.
Freud, S. (1914) 'On narcissism: an introduction', *S.E., Vol. 14*. London: The Hogarth Press, pp. 67–102.
Freud, S. (1923b) *The Ego and the Id. S.E., Vol. 19*. London: The Hogarth Press, pp. 1–66.
Freud, S. (1930a) *Civilisation and its Discontents, S.E., Vol. 21*. London: the Hogarth Press, pp. 57–146.
Freud, S. (1933a) *New Introductory Lectures on Psycho-analysis., S.E., Vol. 22*. London: The Hogarth Press, p. 65.
Press, J. (2011) 'L'inoubliable, limite de l'analysable' ('The Unforgettable, the limit of the analyzable'), in *Construction en psychanalyse: récupérer le passé ou le réinventer*. Paris: Presses Universitaires de France.
Roussillon, R. (2007) 'Pour une clinique de la théorie', *Psychothérapies*, 27, 1, pp. 1–35.
Segal, H. (1957) 'Notes on symbol formation', *Int. J. Psychoanal.*, 38, pp. 391–97.

Chapter 8

Symbolisation

LUIGI SOLANO

The origin of somatic pathology in relation to symbolisation

My position is that body and mind are not separate entities that may be differentiated from the organism as a whole but are two categories connected to the perspective of the observer: this means that we consider only one substance, endowed with both bodily and mental attributes, which may be specifically assessed via different means (e.g. Magnetic Resonance, a clinical interview). This position, which may be defined as 'non-reductionist monism' coupled with 'epistemological dualism' (Solano, 2010, p. 1450; Solano, 2016, p. 55), was originally expressed by Spinoza (1677), and formally introduced in psychoanalytic psychosomatics by Carla De Toffoli (1991; 2011) and Irène Matthis (2000).

It is not possible, at this point, to posit interactions between two entities that have no existence of their own. We may re-establish a dialectic considering the relationships between different levels of experience of reality, and of processing and storing that experience in memory, provided that each level is considered to entail both a bodily and a mental aspect.

These different levels of experience of reality, mostly emerging as three in number, have received different descriptions and names in various theoretical frameworks; I will try to bring these frameworks in relation to each other, since my position, as will be apparent in my writing, is in favour of finding *common ground* among different psychoanalytic theories, where all are seen as valuable approximations to the unknowable *things in themselves*. I will indicate the three levels of experiencing reality with alphabetical letters in order to avoid any idea of a hierarchical subordination:

Level A: Primary Process, raw primary experience of the thing (Freud); Formlessness (Winnicott, 1971, pp. 33–36; Press, 2013a); beta elements (Bion, 1962); implicit memory (Neuroscience); unformulated experience (Stern, 2003); Non-Symbolic System (Bucci, 1997); formal significants (Press, 2013b).

Level B: alpha function, alpha elements (Bion, 1962); thinking in images (Botella and Botella, 2001); oneiric thought of wakefulness (Ferro, 2002); Non-Verbal Symbolic System (Bucci, 1997).

Level C: Secondary Process (Freud); Apparatus for thinking thoughts (Bion); Verbal Symbolic System (Bucci).

I will generally use Wilma Bucci's formulation (which draws largely from many others) since I find it the most comprehensive on all three levels, and because their double nature, both mental and somatic is clearly specified.

In Bucci's view, the Non-Symbolic System (Level A) includes all that happens in the body, seen not as an inert r*es extensa*, but as endowed with basic emotions, and with organised though non-verbal thinking. The Non-Symbolic System and Symbolic Systems are strongly connected in health through 'referential connections' or 'links' (Bucci, 1997, pp. 178–84): this concept is quite different from the notion of transformation of one element into another, such as in the concepts of mentalisation or the transformation of beta into alpha elements, which involves the disappearance of the former element in favour of the latter, considered as more *developed.*

Formation of referential links, which corresponds to what we generally call symbolisation, is highly dependent on a satisfactory object relationship. Links among systems may be insufficiently formed due to insufficient containment (reverie, holding, attunement) on the caretaker's part, or the links may be subsequently interrupted due to traumatic (acute or chronic) conditions. This disconnection leaves behind a disconnected and therefore *nameless* Non-Symbolic arousal in search of connection and/or direct expression.

This disconnection may be described in classical metapsychological terms as 'a drive life which was imperfectly embodied, which has been cut off from its roots' (Press, 2013b, p. 1). Winnicott spoke of detachment of 'mind' from 'psyche-soma' (Winnicott, 1975, pp. 243–324). *Pensée opératoire* (Marty, de M'Uzan and David, 1963) or *vie opératoire* (Smadja, 2001) may be seen as a thought, or a life, disconnected from its emotional (or drive) basis. Alexithymia may be viewed as similar (Nemiah and Sifneos, 1970; Taylor, Bagby and Parker 1997).

Disconnection may be experienced as dullness, boredom, futility, both in the individual and in people relating to her/him (including the analyst). In other instances, a lack of regulation of Non-Symbolic arousal on the part of the Symbolic Systems may account for the sudden emergence of violent, unexplained emotion, as in panic attacks or in *pavor nocturnus*. Non-Symbolic arousal may find spurious, artificial connections to a symbol (as in phobic or persecutory objects which stand as symbols), leading to mental disorders (such as phobias, paranoid disorders) or acting (e.g. eating disorders, paraphilias, antisocial behaviour, etc.)[1]

If none of these operations take place, somatic illness may ensue (Bucci, 2007; Solano, 2010). Bion expressed a similar view about the fate and effects of untransformed beta elements. In the discussions of our working party, Nick Temple suggested that somatic illness might ensue when individuals fail to reach the paranoid-schizoid position (where they might find a persecutory content for a disconnected and nameless Non-Symbolic arousal). In this framework, somatic pathology might be connected with the 'contiguous-autistic position', proposed by Ogden (Ogden, 1989), as developmentally antedating the paranoid-schizoid position. The emergence of disconnected Non-Symbolic arousal in any form is greatly facilitated by its resonance with the present life situations of the individual.

We end up, therefore, with a vision of somatic disorders that are not caused by something in the mind which finds its expression in the body as in hysterical conversion disorders.[2] Instead, we envisage a body (a Non-Symbolic System) reacting to problems concerning the individual's relationship with his/her world with little or no connection to mental (symbolic) processing, which could otherwise regulate and give expression to the reaction.

A possible progressive/activating value of somatic symptoms

A possible developmental and progressive value of somatic symptoms was proposed by Winnicott in his work, 'The Mind and Its Relationship to the Psyche-Soma' (Winnicott, 1949), where somatic symptoms are described as an attempt to 'draw the psyche from the mind back to its original intimate association with the soma' (1975, p. 254). In other words, we may view a somatic symptom, besides being a witness to disconnection, as the Non-Symbolic, first expression of an item of content that had until then not found any possibility of expression.

An echo of this position may be found in Smadja (2001), where he notices how the appearance of a somatic symptom may give relief to a patient, as if, in the absence of available psychic objects, somatic organs and functions may be optimal. This last set of notations may suggest the existence of possible dissociations, not only between systems but within the Non-Symbolic system itself (Bucci, 2007); in this sense, a somatic symptom could be viewed as a way of overcoming dissociation.

Symbolic meaning of somatic symptoms

In the model proposed, where somatic symptoms arise from Non-Symbolic arousal, the presence from the beginning of symbolic meaning is by definition excluded. This contrasts with a model of somatisation, which may hold true for conversion hysteria where the body is used simply as a place (a stage) for representing emotions or conflicts which were perceived but rejected by the mind.[3]

But it also contrasts with authors such as Groddeck, Chiozza or Garma who believed in an autonomous body language: they postulate a universal, a priori, symbolic meaning for different somatic symptoms.

If we think about the body as having a language, this does not necessarily mean a symbolic language. In the same way that we do not believe that dreams have a universal, definite meaning a priori, but that their meaning may be constructed in analysis, symbolic meanings of the body's expression may be constructed in the analytic relationship. This position was supported by Carla De Toffoli (2011) and mostly accepted in our group. Bérangère de Senarclens wrote: 'Similar to the way the infant expresses its bodily and psychic needs to his mother, the patient's symptoms or repetitive actings express a strong demand for symbolisation from the analyst . . . A call for comprehension, for meaning and containment, even if it is not there "a priori"' (De Senarclens, 2013, p. 3); Jacques Press also wrote of the 'potential symbolic value' of somatic symptoms (Press, 2014, p. 2). A clinical point to be stressed about the construction of meaning in analysis is the importance of remaining for a long time at the Non-Symbolic (concrete, sensory) level with the patient – where the object may be used in a 'sensory basis' rather than an 'object basis' – without premature attempts at 'translation' into symbolic terms (Racalbuto, 1994, pp. 8–13).

Cate: initial presentation

Cate's difficulty in symbolisation is apparent from her first utterance, the message left on the answering machine: 'The name she gave wasn't audible and I couldn't make out which one was her first name and which one her surname'. The misunderstanding at the door at the time of her first appointment also suggests an enactment communicating something Cate is incapable of expressing in words. The fantasy that no help exists for her hints at the content that is expressed in the two episodes: if no help exists, it is useless to state one's name clearly, it is useless to ring the bell, or to ring it carefully. Lack of symbolisation also shows up in her narrative about her romantic relationships: 'My relationships last two and a half years and then I leave'. She does not know why.

In the session, we witness different expressions of what the author calls 'bodily anxiety' (which we might also call Non-Symbolic arousal): crying with only partial awareness of the reasons; moving backwards and forwards in her armchair rubbing her hands at the same time. Outside the session, Cate reports different ways of sedating, or of discharging bodily anxiety through acting: use of alcohol, going out alone to bars at nights.

Continuing the interview, Cate gives us hints of how the disconnection between bodily anxiety and symbolic representations came to be. A felt lack of containment and of listening on the part of her mother may have prevented the formation of links between what I called Level A and the other two levels. Links appear also to be *crossed out* in anger: 'As she feels that she doesn't exist for her mother she eliminates her intrapsychically'. Later in the interview, her *crossing out links* – specifically in terms of visual symbols – emerges in the dream where the paintings in an art gallery disappear.

The importance of physical illness and the ensuing emotions, as a first effort towards reconnection, is described by the analyst as 'a movement of narcissistic reinvestment'. Fotis Bobos carefully investigates the presence of important events just before the appearance of cancer. In fact, he does find a convergent set of events: reduction of income, serious problems with her boyfriend, her son's reduced needs for continuous presence and care, changes in her body because of ageing. In the presence of insufficient connections with symbolic systems, the ensuing bodily (non-symbolic) anxiety finds expression through physical illness.

Evolution through analysis

The first session reported from the third year of analytic work starts with 'happiness working on the farm with her plants' and 'feeling lonely and deciding to meet her boyfriend'. Physical symptoms and physical expressions (crying, drinking, moving in the chair, rubbing hands) are substituted with feelings. This not only allows for the expression and regulation of Level A phenomena but may have other useful effects: happiness builds up the cohesion of self and promotes self-esteem; loneliness stimulates purposeful and not evacuative action. Cate is capable of keeping quiet for more than five minutes, which possibly means that she is thinking, that she does not need to immediately evacuate emotions she has not yet understood (translated to feelings). Her effort towards symbolisation is shown in her attempt to find symbols (though probably spurious ones) for her sense of rejection from her mother: 'her mother wanted her to be a boy; her mother wanted her and her brother to be a couple'.

In the second session, we learn that Cate has stopped smoking pot: she needs less sedation, since her anxiety has found ways of expression. The dream of the guardian angel shows a greatly improved internal representation of a relationship with a caring figure. This is confirmed by the expression of care towards the analyst: 'please do not get sick'. The dream where sessions are portrayed as sleeping and sitting loosely in armchairs, seems to point to the importance of a non-verbal, Level A, Non-Symbolic exchange (Racalbuto, 1994).

Jasmine: initial presentation

Different to Cate, Jasmine at the beginning shows little signs of disconnection or dysregulation, except possibly the sense of being rushed and in a hurry, as if the need for analysis had not found its way into symbolisation/consciousness in due time, and only emerged abruptly at the last minute. She gives an 'articulate and rather touching account of her life', to the point that the analyst wonders about her motivation for seeking analysis. At the same time, though, she has the sense of 'something quite troubling and inaccessible'. In the second consultation (on two occasions), the analyst is aware of a selective incapacity to identify a specific emotion (worry), suggesting some disconnection between Non-symbolic and Symbolic systems. This impression is present in the countertransferential idea of preventive reasons for psychoanalysis.

For a moment, the patient signals a clear problem: a sense of futility, as if she had become aware of a disconnection with her most basic needs and emotions. The analyst formulates the thought of having identified with an object 'who considered her self-sufficient and certainly not in need of anything coming from the other', and that this might have caused the analyst's feeling that the patient had no need for analysis. This message from the object might have contributed to her disconnection from her basic needs. Towards the end of the session, Jasmine's emotions show inadequate regulation at a more symbolic, cognitive level (Level C): she speaks of 'desperation', of 'outbursts of rage', of 'almost compulsion to undo my life in fury' with no proportion to real life events.

On the eve of her analysis, Jasmine develops acute abdominal pain. In the theoretical framework proposed, this may be viewed as a first, non-symbolic expression of a traumatic memory, which is reactivated by the patient accepting entrance into a helping relationship. 'A leap of the somatic into her psychic world' is the pregnant formulation given by Marina Perris, which I perfectly agree with. I would add that this formulation is different from others found in Marina's paper such as 'somatisation' or 'acting-in in the body', or (later on) 'somatic regression', which suggest the opposite route – from mind to body – and which I consider to be only a feature of hysterical symptoms. Apart from this episode, however, expression of Non-Symbolic arousal remains very poor for several years, a situation which I see as at high risk of giving rise to sudden violent acting or episodes of severe disease in the case of the failure of her defences (Solano, 2015). In this sense, being in analysis was indeed a very effective form of *prevention*.

Jasmine's memories of her relationship with her mother confirm the hypothesis of a deficit in caring, in attunement, in reverie, in holding, and more generally in capacities of connecting Level A experiences with symbolic levels. The mother is described by Jasmine as not expecting her, as being more devoted to her older sisters and brother. Jasmine 'had no memory of the mother's physical affection', and this feeling was more present and painful when she was ill: she felt her mother 'could not stand' her being ill. Lack of acceptance of illness, and probably of negative emotions, may well be linked with Jasmine's difficulty in expressing her needs in any way, including somatic symptoms.

Evolution in analysis

After six years of analysis, Jasmine is becoming capable of expressing negative feelings (discontent and disappointment) towards the analyst, possibly deriving from her early experiences with her mother. Discontent and disappointment are also enacted in the 'non-affair' with Mr K, where she ends up feeling sexually aroused without an adequate fulfilment. Parallel to this, the growth of cysts in her breast enacts in the analytic relationship a situation where death anxieties are present and strongly signalled, but the object is very seldom present. The analyst is brought to share her distress concretely (as in the Bionian concept of O link).

At the same time, Jasmine seems very keen on exploring whether, in the sessions, when the analyst is present, things may this time go differently, whether she may receive adequate attention and sharing of her often deadly distress ('she was almost ill with anxiety and pain in her breast') and for her cry for help. Arousal and ensuing frustration emerge clearly in the 'erotic' dream with Mr K, and in the episode with her cousin, together with the hope that, this time, the analyst will 'look' at her breasts. The analyst finds herself in the countertransference feeling the mother's dismissal, a strong dislike for the image of a baby feeding at the breast. She can elaborate this image, returning it to the patient in interpretation, and so proceed towards symbolisation, a 'restoration of representation of psychic events'.

In the words of the analyst, 'split-off early traumatic experiences returned to be worked through. In that first instance, as there were no words for them, these experiences were 'spoken of' in the language of the body'. The meaning of these symptoms, in the model I have proposed, is constructed *in* the analytic situation, and is not present from the start. Similarly, I would rather think that the possibility of working in the preconscious and in the representational field is reached, not returned to, since fruitful work on representations is possible only when these represent substantially what goes on at a non-representational level.

FOTIS BOBOS

Introduction

'In the beginning was the Deed', concludes Freud at the end of *Totem and Taboo* in 1913 (Freud, 1913, p. 161). He compares children to primitive men, where the distinction between thinking and doing is absent, and their psychic reality is equal to what he calls their factual reality (i.e. primitive men actually did what they intended to do). Children and primitive men are uninhibited: thought passes directly into action, and the deed is a substitute for thought. In contrast, neurotics are, above all, inhibited in their actions: for them, the thought is a complete substitute for the deed. Two years earlier, Freud (1911) suggested that postponement of action enables thought processes to develop through the representation of ideas. Thinking is essentially an experimental, hypothetical kind of act with a smaller quantity of cathexis and less discharge of it than action.

With regard to the relationship between acting and speech, Green argues that when the transference of all psychic elements into speech is obstructed then the excitations discharged find an outlet by acting in the external world or in the body: 'Acting out is the external counterpart to the psychosomatic acting in. It has the same value in expelling psychic reality' (Green, 1975, p. 6). Hence, acting out to a certain extent is an alternative way of maintaining a psychosomatic equilibrium (Donnet, 2005), preventing psychosomatic acting in, which thereby protects the body.

As we refer to language symbolism, it could be useful to explore the meaning of the word symbol; the term derives from the Greek word *σύμβολο*, which means token or sign. It is a compound word from the preposition *συν*, which means 'together', and *βολή* which means 'a throwing, a casting'. Campbell defines the symbol as an energy evoking and directing agent (1969, p. 143). The symbol has the meaning of something that stands for something else: of something visible that by association or connection represents something else that is invisible.

Symbolism and primary and secondary processes

According to Freud's topographical model, symbolisation takes place at the preconscious level through the secondary processes, which relate word representations to thing representations. With the primary symbolisation processes at the unconscious level (Roussillon, 1999), the first psychic material in the form of mnemonic perceptive traces of things are organised and transformed into thing representations at which point they can accede to the preconscious level. The classic psychoanalytic work relies on the secondary symbolisation processes: language symbolisation. The analyst works on the psychic thing representations which have already been modified by the primary symbolisation processes, rather than on the raw perceptive experience of the thing itself. In the structural model, the Id includes a large part of the unconscious and goes beyond it, so that it is to a great extent open to stimuli coming from the body. Primary symbolisation concerns the body itself and constitutes the grounds of the ego formation, which is above all 'ultimately derived from bodily sensations' (Freud, 1923, p. 26).

The analyst's symbolisation function

In psychosomatic states, our clinical observation of insufficiency in psychic processes leads us to the view that the patient has experienced anew a traumatic situation, which reactivates the primary one. The lack of available unconscious representations that could be mobilised, leads to the hypothesis of deficient forms of thing representations at the level of primary symbolisation processes. Consequently, we could assume that in these cases analytic work would constitute first of all work at the level of primary symbolisation, a mentalisation process made by the analyst, based on acting out (towards the analyst) and/or acting in the body (somatisation) of the patient.

Regarding the therapeutic attitude and technique, the majority of analysts from different psychoanalytic currents of thought agree in attributing the maternal object function to the analyst in treating traumatised patients, i.e. those who are isolated from the external object and cut off from their bodily experiences. In these cases, we cannot but think of Winnicott's well known phrase: 'There is no such thing as an infant', meaning, of course, that whenever one finds an infant one finds maternal care, and without maternal care there would be no infant' (Winnicott, 1960, p. 587).

In particular, the analysts of the Paris Psychosomatics School suggest that work with psychosomatic patients benefits from face-to-face seating instead of the couch. In addition, placing the patient in the armchair provides him/her with some freedom of movement, which can be perceptible to the analyst. Bodily movements express what has not been sufficiently symbolised and therefore cannot be verbally expressed. These bodily expressions correspond to and constitute precursor forms of adult thinking. Mobility and acting, which are addressed to the analyst and are actualised within the analytic relationship, comprise a privileged form of manifesting experiences that are excluded to some extent from psychic elaboration.

In the same train of thought, I think that Fain's concept of 'The censorship of the lover' (Fain, 1971) can provide us with particularly useful thoughts regarding the analyst's functioning. According to Fain, 'The censorship of the lover' pertains to the double role of the primary object. As a caring mother, she is present, receives, gives meaning to, and satisfies the baby's needs. As a woman-lover, she is absent, seeking to satisfy her own erotic, sexual wishes with her lover. Fain suggests that on the one hand 'The mother's cathexis of the newborn is accompanied by a narcissistic retreat that extends to maternalising the environment' (Fain, 1971, p. 340). On the other hand, 'A woman survives somewhere . . . Thus, the representation of a hallucinatory satisfaction of the other's desire, prefiguring a later primal scene, is depicted outside the mothering environment' (Fain, 1971, p. 340).

Accordingly, we might postulate that in his countertransference the analyst also assumes the double role of presence and absence analogous to the double role and function of the primary object: on the one hand, the analyst is present with the patient in the session, being attentive, giving meaning to stimuli, and becoming a protective shield function for his patient. On the other hand, the analyst is absent from the session in order to satisfy his own libidinal desires with another. These two roles reach their peak at the end of the session which is imposed on the patient by the analyst and can be seen as the imposition of a kind of *censorship* (the censorship of the lover, i.e. the analyst leaves the patient for someone else). During the session the analyst is concerned with the feelings of helplessness, thereby he is functioning as an 'ethical subject' (Chetrit-Vatine, 2014). Through his absence in his desire for another object, elements of the absent erotic other are set in motion and constructed in the patient's inner world. Having cathected the gratifying mother-analyst, the patient starts to cathect the analyst's desire for the absent third; the experiences of the early triangulation, as a precursor to the organisation of the primal scene, are reinvested. The rather satisfactory alternations of the analyst's functioning presence and absence reinforces the patient's capability for representation.

Roussillon, among other analysts, has provided various interesting ideas about the analytic work on symbolisation (Roussillon, 1999). The analyst's interventions include both verbal and nonverbal content which convey meanings. The nonverbal audio-sensory stimuli of the analyst's interpretations are determined by his style of expressing emotions, e.g. his tone of voice, and the timing and rhythm of his utterances, etc. The verbal content consists of the analyst's constructions based on his countertransference feelings, linked with scenarios which he creates by accepting all verbal and non-verbal stimuli coming from his inner world and from the patient's.

The flexibility of the analyst's constructions is very significant in order to avoid reactivation of traumatic zones; there is always the risk that the patient might experience the analyst's interventions as actions that induce a new trauma. Moreover, the analyst's flexibility of construction creates the possibility of more than one and even contradictory meanings, opening pathways to the emotional reinforcement and organisation of thing representations.

The analyst uses his/her perceptual image of the patient's bodily movements or acting and links them with potential meanings in order to symbolise these movements. Perhaps the language that the analyst uses corresponds better to *tongue* rather than to *language* in English. The two words derive from the same Proto-Indo-European linguistic root, but they differ significantly with regard to body proximity and thus meaning. The word *tongue* means the fleshy muscular organ in the mouth used for tasting, licking, swallowing, and articulating speech; but in the sense of *mother or native tongue*, the word tongue refers to the *first language*, revealing the close bodily connection between *tongue* and the primary object.

In keeping the word *language* for the secondary symbolisation processes, one could say that both the acting body that discharges the tension towards the object, and the suffering body that discharges tension to the psychosomatic unit, do not convey symbolic meaning and therefore do not speak. They search for the symbolism that emerges through the relationship with the object in a way that is similar to the infant who expresses its bodily and psychic needs to his mother who will satisfy them in an adequate way. The need for symbolisation underlines what has not yet been sufficiently integrated. The repetitive compulsory acting imposed upon the analyst's mind expresses the strong 'demand for representation', and as Aisentein perspicuously suggests: 'the first demand for representation is that which is addressed by the body, of which it could be said that it is a demand for translation addressed to the mind'. (Aisenstein, 2013, p. 177).

The two clinical cases

Cate

Cate's initial interviews, characterised mostly by her intense motor discharge and extreme irritability at environmental stimuli, manifest a state of being alert and helpless. This behaviour had an important impact on a countertransferential level. I had the feeling that I somehow had to give an answer by adopting a more active stance. My aim was to make my living existence perceptible to Cate by receiving verbal and non-verbal stimuli and trying to selectively put some of these into words. I think that such an attitude could create protection from the overwhelming, disastrous transferential storm that makes Cate, as well as me, disappear into nothingness.

The debacle of the closed door, which Cate perceived as a great injustice regardless of the reason, was an additional factor that set me in motion to display my emotional availability to her. At the same time, I felt the need to cathect her body, so I expressed an interest in the physical illness of her cancer – which was her main motive for asking for help – by making certain hypothetical links between the illness and the psychic contents she projected. I think that my 'seductive' words apropos of the tissues, reveal my openness to her life perspective in contrast to her projective fear of me being unavailable. Her bursting into tears is an indication of discharge from a depressive state, which cannot yet be organised and psychically represented. My intervention that links the feeling of emptiness with 'crossing out' her mother affects her and brings out the screen memory of her father's traumatic abandonment. It seems that the father has been more maternal figure than her mother.

In the sessions of the third year, the analytic work focuses on issues of being rejected by others and denial of the transference relationship. I think that my intervention linking her acting out – her searching for my receptiveness during summer vacations – and her projection of being rejected by me in the sessions, induces symbolisation process; Cate's feeling of rejection leads her to the thought of having been rejected as a female by her mother, bringing back the conflictual issue of her sexual identity.

In the next session, the second dream seems to be an associative interpretation of the first one. The dream work starts with the fear of contact with a threatening object, which later on takes the form of the guardian angel's caress. It reminds me of the common representation of the caring mother as guardian angel during the young child's sleep. This care is also symbolised by the image of a kiss on the cheek by the caring mother-analyst at the moment the dream ends. Nevertheless, in the real time of the session, the narration of the dream causes emotional arousal, expressed in the form of physical excitement which underlines the fear of punishment imposed on her by me, and/or a punishment I may undergo by her. As a mother Cate takes care of and protects her son, and through a role reversal, she functions as an encouraging mother to her parents.

Jasmine

By the end of Jasmine's sixth year in analysis, we could say that a splitting process is reactivated in the psychosomatic unity of the patient. On the one hand, Jasmine's hypochondriac fears about her breast cysts threaten both the analyst and herself; on the other hand, her erotic feelings find a release through a lateral transference in her relationship with Mr. K, but without any bodily contact.

The experience of being psychically paralysed seems to be an identification with the mother; an active repetition of her memory of her paralysed mother, who held her baby tight during the fire. I think that the way in which Jasmine constantly brings her body close to the analyst reveals an attempt to hold the analyst tight. Moreover, it would be better for Jasmine to share her agonising and torturous fate with the analyst, rather than live without a mother-analyst. The new somatic symptom of the recurrent cysts, followed by the dread of cancer, intensifies the vital need to be alive by *catching* the analyst.

I think that the analyst's interpretation of the missing session as a condensation of the conflict between two opposite forces – both leaving the analyst and needing the analyst – has great symbolic value. Jasmine's image of grabbing and squeezing the analyst's arm/breast, and raising her arms to show her two fists, expresses her inner desire: a mirroring relationship with the mother-analyst which involves touching each other violently. Jasmine's desire condenses the closely interconnected sexual and aggressive components of a baby's motor movement, a primitive form of physical affection.

I think that the transferential dream constitutes the result of her symbolic elaboration of the rest of the previous session; that is, her feelings of guilt linked with her desire to look and be looked at, to touch and be touched by the analyst. Working on the transference has mostly been complemented by the work on countertransference. The analyst creates a scene in which the patient feels humiliated by the analyst's unreciprocated love and therefore becomes melancholic. We could suppose that the somatic functional symptoms, as well as the benign physical symptom form a substitute for the organisation of melancholy, although traces of melancholic feelings appear from the beginning.

Commentary

NICK TEMPLE

The two authors of this chapter, Fotis Bobos and Luigi Solano, present contrasting but related views on the role of symbolisation in psychosomatic states, which are made clearer by their discussion of the clinical material in the two cases. They both agree that the analyst's role in developing symbolic capacity is crucial and is demonstrated in the improvement shown by the patients Cate and Jasmine in the later stages of their treatment.

Luigi Solano uses Bucci's formulation on symbolisation which outlines three levels of mental functioning. (1) a non-symbolic system; (2) a non-verbal symbolic system; and (3) a verbal symbolic system.

In this view, somatic symptoms occur when symbolic operations have failed to take place. Luigi makes the point that somatic disorders are not caused by something in the mind finding expression in the body (as in hysterical conversion disorders), but the body reacting to problems in the patient's inner world with little or no connection to symbolic functioning. He refers to Winnicott's observation 'that draws the psyche from the mind back to its original intimate association with the soma.' Luigi's comment that the failed movement from the paranoid-schizoid to the depressive position results in somatic illness is similar to Segal's (1957) view that symbolic capacity depends on reaching the depressive position in relation to the object.

Luigi also quotes Smajda's view that the appearance of a somatic symptom may give relief to a patient, as if in the absence of available psychic objects, somatic organs and functions may be employed. In Luigi's model, where somatic symptoms are linked to non-symbolic arousal, the presence of symbolic meaning is by definition excluded. This is in contrast to the model of somatisation which may hold true for conversion hysteria, where the body is used as a place for representing emotions or conflicts which were perceived but rejected by the mind.

A key point that Luigi makes is that non-symbolic and symbolic systems are connected. The formation of the links necessary for symbolisation are highly dependent on a satisfactory object relationship, and these links may be insufficiently formed or disrupted by poor containment or damaged by traumatic experience.

Both authors emphasise the point that the relationship with the analyst plays a key role in developing the patient's capacity for symbolisation and results in a slow move away from somatic symptoms. This is demonstrated in the material from both patients Cate and Jasmine, who develop an increased capacity for symbolic thinking in the later sessions of analytic work. Luigi makes the point that with Cate the improved capacity for symbolisation has brought with it a greater capacity for making distinctions between self and object and between objects.

Luigi stresses the clinical risks in the analysis of premature attempts of translation in symbolic terms; there is a need to remain at the non-symbolic level for a sufficient time. He points out that symbolic language may be constructed in the analytic relationship in the same way that the meaning of dreams is constructed in the analytic work. In this respect, it is interesting that the appearance of dreams related to the transference relationship can occur when there is a move away from physical symptoms. This shows the development of the capacity to represent the transference relationship and the internal world symbolically.

Fotis Bobos refers to Freud's observation in *Totem and Taboo* where he compares children to primitive men for whom the sharp contrast between thinking and doing is absent, and here he suggests that psychosomatic symptoms might be regarded as a form of action. This is in contrast to neurotics who are above all inhibited in their actions, and thought is a complete substitute for the deed. Fotis refers to Green who goes one step further in saying that 'acting out is the external counterpart to psychosomatic acting in, it has the same value in expelling psychic reality'. This view suggests that psychosomatic acting in is a defensive step to avoid psychic reality, just as acting out is. In this sense, Green suggests that the symbols representing psychic reality have been expelled. Here, Fotis's perspective is in contrast with Luigi's view that symbolisation has not developed and must be constructed during the analytic work.

Fotis also differentiates primary symbolic processes from secondary symbolisation which is used in classical psychoanalytical work. The classical work of analysis is based on symbolisation of language, whereas primary symbolisation is related to the body. In this sense, Fotis makes the key point that 'tongue' represents the primary bodily symbol, whereas 'language' represents the secondary symbol based on words. It is interesting to note whether primary symbolisation would equate to the symbolic equation described by Segal (1957) as a primitive symbolic process.

Fotis emphasises the analysts symbolising function with the patient, and he relates this to the analyst's function as the maternal object in traumatised patients. He refers here to Roussillon's thoughts on symbolisation which require the analyst to put his constructions from the countertransference into words via interpretation. Fotis also makes the point that the analyst must avoid reactivating traumatic areas in this work. However, he points out that the analytic work may result in the patient experiencing a new trauma which reactivates the primary traumatic situation. This is evident in his discussion of Jasmine where the negative feelings are initially concealed by idealisation but are later expressed through hypochondriacal fears associated with the functional somatic symptoms.

Fotis agrees with Luigi that a central part of the analytic work will be developing the patient's capacity to symbolise, in line with Roussillon's view. They may differ on the point of whether they are defining an absence of symbolisation or a difficulty of secondary symbolisation in words and language. It would be interesting to discuss the question of to what extent the somatic symptoms can function as a defensive organisation against primitive anxieties, in line with Green's point about somatic symptoms avoiding psychic reality. This raises the question of the persecutory nature of the relationship with the internal objects, which might be defended against. The point that both authors make that a key role of the analyst is to support the symbolic function in the patient, can be regarded as the containing function offered by a good analytic relationship in working through primitive anxieties.

Notes

1 The relentless search for meaning on the part of 'nameless' Non-Symbolic arousal may be compared to Roussillon's notion of a 'compulsion to integrate' (Roussillon, 2015).
2 This position is accurately illustrated by Nick Temple in Chapter 7: 'The psychic conflict is *transformed into a physical symptom*' (my italics). He also uses Aisenstein's concept of *acting in the body.*
3 Jacques Press considers symbolic meaning to be present (a priori) in a continuum linked to the degree of disorganisation from hysterical symptoms to severe organic disease (Press, 2014). I can only agree with a position favouring a dimensional approach over rigid categories.

References

Aisenstein, M. (2013) 'Drive, representation and the demands of representation', in H. Levine, G. Reed and D. Scarfone (eds), *The Unrepresented States and the Construction of Meaning: Clinical and Theoretical Contributions*. London: Karnac, pp. 175–88.

Bion, W.R. (1962) *Learning from Experience*. London: Heinemann.

Botella, C. and Botella S. (2001) *La figurabilité psychique*. Paris/Neuchâtel: Delachaux & Niestlé [*The Work of Psychic Figurability: Mental States Without Representation*. London: Routledge, 2004].

Bucci, W. (1997) *Psychoanalysis and Cognitive Science. A Multiple Code Theory*. New York: Guilford Press.

Bucci, W. (2007) 'Dissociation from the perspective of multiple code theory, Part I: Psychological roots and implications for the psychoanalytic treatment', *Contemporary Psychoanalysis*, 43, pp. 165–84.

Campbell, J. (1969) *Flight of the Wild Gander: The Symbol without Meaning*. Novato, CA: New World Library, 2002.

Chetrit-Vatine, V. (2014) *The Ethical Seduction of the Analytic Situation: The Feminine-Maternal Origins of Responsibility for the Other*. London: Karnac.

De Senarclens, B. (2013) 'The meaning of the symptom. Communication to Members of the Working Party in Psychosomatics', European Psychoanalytic Federation.

De Toffoli, C. (1991) 'L'invenzione di un pensiero dal versante somatico della relazione', *Rivista di Psicoanalisi*, 38, pp. 563–97.

De Toffoli, C. (2011) 'The living body in the psychoanalytic experience', *Psychoanalytic Quarterly*, 80, pp. 595–618.

Donnet, J.L. (2005) *The Analyzing Situation*. London: Karnac, 2009.

Fain, M. (1971) 'The prelude to fantasmatic life', in D. Birksted-Breen, S. Flanders, and A. Gibault (eds), (2010), *Reading French Psychoanalysis*. London: Routledge, pp. 338–54.

Ferro, A. (2002) *Fattori di malattia, fattori di guarigione*. Milan: Cortina. [Seeds of illness, seeds of recovery]. London: Routledge, 2004.

Freud, S. (1911) 'Formulations on the two principles of mental functioning', *S.E., Vol. 12*. London: The Hogarth Press, pp. 213–26.

Freud, S. (1913) *Totem and Taboo, S.E., Vol. 13*. London: The Hogarth Press, pp. 1–162.

Freud, S. (1923) *The Ego and the Id, S.E., Vol. 19*. London: The Hogarth Press, pp. 1–66.

Green, A. (1975) 'The analyst, symbolization and absence in the analytic setting', *Int. J. Psychoanal.*, 56, pp. 1–22.

Marty, P., de M'Uzan, M. and David, C. (1963) *L'investigation psychosomatique*. Paris: Presses Universitaires de France.

Matthis, I. (2000) 'Sketch for a metapsychology of affect', *Int. J. Psychoanal.*, 81, pp. 215–27.

Nemiah, J.C. and Sifneos, P.E. (1970) 'Affect and fantasy in patients with psychosomatic disorders', in O.W. Hill (ed.), *Modern Trends in Psychosomatic Medicine*. London: Butterworths, pp. 26–34.

Ogden, T.H. (1989) 'On the concept of an autistic-contiguous position', *Int. J. Psychoanal.*, 70, pp. 127–40.

Press, J. (2013a) 'Formlessness, the intimate, the unknown processes of transformation and the object. Formlessness: deformation, transformation', 26th Annual Conference of the European Psychoanalytic Federation. Basel, March 21–24.

Press, J. (2013b) 'Some Lines of Research', Communication to Members of the Working Party.

Press, J. (2014) 'Ruptures, somatisations and countertransference. Intervention to the Panel "Ruptures in the outside world, rupture in the psychesoma: Trauma and somatic illness"'. Ruptures: The 27th Annual Conference of the European Psychoanalytic Federation, Turin, April 10–13.

Racalbuto, A. (1994) *Tra il fare e il dire: L'esperienza dell'inconscio e del non verbale in psicoanalisi*. Milan: Cortina.

Roussillon, R. (2015) 'Foundations and processes in the psychoanalytic encounter', Conference, La Relazione Analitica. Bologna, 14–15 February 2015.

Roussillon, R. (1999) *Primitive Agony and Symbolization*. London: Karnac, 2011.

Segal, H. (1957) 'Notes on symbol formation', *Int. J. Psychoanal.*, 38, pp. 391–97.

Smadja, C. (2001) *La vie opératoire: Etudes psychoanalytiques*. Paris: Presses Universitaires de France.

Solano, L. (2010) 'Some thoughts between body and mind in the light of Wilma Bucci's multiple code theory', *International Journal of Psychoanalysis*, 91, pp. 1445–64.

Solano, L. (2015) 'Beyond symptoms: Towards an assessment based on level of integration', 28th European Psychoanalytic Federation Conference: Too much – not enough, Stockholm, March 21–24, pp. 33–34.

Solano, L. (2016) 'Al di là di Cartesio: Riflessioni sul corpomente', *Rivista di Psicoanalisi*, 62, pp. 49–72.

Spinoza, B. (1677) *Ethica. Part III*. Prop. II.

Stern, D.B. (2003) *Unformulated Experience: From Dissociation to Imagination in Psychoanalysis*. London: Routledge.

Taylor, G.J., Bagby, R.M. and Parker, J.M.A. (1997) *Disorders of Affect Regulation*. Cambridge: Cambridge University Press.

Winnicott, D.W. (1949) 'Mind and its relation to the psyche-soma', *British Journal of Medical Psychology*, 27, pp. 201–209, 1954] [Reprinted in *Through Pediatrics to Psychoanalysis*. London: The Hogarth Press and the Institute of Psychoanalysis, 1975].

Winnicott, D.W. (1971) *Playing and Reality*. London: Tavistock Publications.

Winnicott, D.W. (1960) 'The theory of the parent-infant relationship', *Int. J. Psychoanal.*, 41, pp. 585–95.

Chapter 9

Defence mechanisms and levels of integration

LUIGI SOLANO

I would slightly reformulate the question posed by the title of this chapter in the following terms: to what extent are health and diseases (including physical ones) linked to defence mechanisms, and to what extent are they linked to a failure in transformation or integration due to deficiencies in primary care?

In the history of psychoanalysis, we find different positions on this topic. The Paris Psychosomatic School's definition of *pensée opératoire* (Marty, de M'Uzan and David, 1963) seems to refer to a low capacity for integration, in the sense of a low capacity on the part of thought to integrate drive energy. Similarly, Smadja's *vie opératoire* is seen as the effect of disconnection – between body and mind, between Id and ego, which may lead to a 'de-regulation' of physiological functions (Smadja, 2001).

Other contemporary authors also view somatic disease as linked to a disconnection between non-symbolic and symbolic systems (Bucci, 1997), or between a physiological and a cognitive-experiential level of emotion (Taylor, Bagby and Parker, 1997): this latter formulation was proposed as the structural determinant of alexithymia. Both Bucci and Taylor attribute this disconnection (or dissociation or lack of integration) to traumatic or deficient care situations. (A view of somatic illness as associated with disconnection among systems or levels is described extensively in my contribution to Chapter 8.)

Winnicott, in his well-known paper 'Psycho-Somatic Illness in its Positive and Negative Aspects', speaks of psychosomatic illness as due to 'dissociations' or a 'split' in the patient (Winnicott, 1966, p. 510). This points to lack of integration, and towards the end of the paper this is attributed to 'maternal failure which leaves the infant without the essentials for the operation of the maturational processes' (Winnicott, 1966, p. 515); the achievement of psychosomatic integration is seen as the aim of treatment. In other parts of the paper, however, Winnicott seems to refer to *defences* leading to this situation: 'This illness state in the patient is itself a defence organisation with very powerful determinants . . . the forces at work in the patient are tremendously strong' (Winnicott, 1966, p. 510). He writes, 'Many patients do not split their medical care into two; the split is into many fragments' (Winnicott, 1966, p. 510). Patients with multiple dissociations also exploit the natural splits in the medical profession such as: medical/surgical, family physician/specialists, psychiatric/psychotherapeutic, etc. In other words, 'the patient's pathological splitting' extends to 'the environmental provision'; this 'separates psyche-care from soma-care' (Winnicott, 1966, p. 511).[1] In a different way, Joyce McDougall's notion of *désaffectation*, of detaching affect from experience, appears mainly as a form of defence (McDougall, 1989).

Bion's position is clearly articulated: on the one hand, a *defective* alpha function may cause an accumulation of beta elements, leading to damage in bodily functions (Bion, 1962). At some points, however, more than a deficit, Bion appears to postulate that beta elements may be (defensively, we might say) *rejected* by the alpha function when there are too many of them or when they are too painful (Grotstein, 2008, p. 60). Here, the alpha function may also be (defensively) attacked and damaged, and even reversed in its direction, in order to avoid painful feelings and frustration.

A synthesis of deficit and defensive aspects that I have found very fruitful is proposed by James Grotstein in his account of determinants for highly alexithymic conditions: a lack of containment, a lack of attunement, any kind of failure in primary relationships leads to a failure in processing proto-affects and in translating emotions into feelings (Grotstein, 1997).[2] For such subjects, affects remain at a very primitive level (beta elements in Bion, symmetry in Matte Blanco, formlessness in Winnicott). When confronted with the danger of being submerged in an avalanche of primitive affects, *the subject may organise general and massive defences* against affects. At this point, we might view the *split* or *dissociation* as linked to traumas or failures in primary relationships, which then become the *cause* of the subsequent defence. Moreover, the two components, dissociation and defences, may be deeply intertwined. At any rate, it appears very difficult, and possibly unhelpful, to exclude the contribution of either an integration deficit, or a defensive component, in the pathogenesis of somatic disorders.

Cate

The initial episode with the doorbell can easily be seen as the enactment of a disconnection (the analyst also appears in this position): possibly it is not so important to define whether it was the analyst who did not hear the doorbell or the patient who did not ring it (or rang it very briefly or did not ring it again); the field, we might say, portrays a disconnection. Cate continues to talk about a 'relationship that hasn't existed', which the analyst feels and interprets also as a fantasy of 'non-existent help' in the relationship with him. He also feels drawn to 'make a link' between the presence of a somatic symptom and the feeling of a non-existent relationship; that is, to promote integration.

Disconnection is also evident in several instances where Cate appears to be unaware of the reasons for her actions: 'My relations last two and a half years and then I leave'. Her constant wish to leave her present boyfriend is mostly unexplained, while her staying in the relationship (in spite of constant strong feelings against the man) is also unexplained. Cate describes herself as 'frozen' and coming to life as 'thawing'. Rage and provocativeness (at school) also appear to bring about some integration. Lack of integration, as described in the theories reported above, may be attributed to lack of adequate containment, which in the patient's words appears as a feeling of being neglected, of her mother's preference for her brother, etc.

Cate, however, also shows active defences at work. In her participation in group psychotherapy she takes on a position of counsellor for newcomers, thus projecting her needs and emotions. She is also aware of 'crossing out' people who might arouse strong emotions in her – her mother and analyst included. 'Freezing' may also be seen as an active defence and is so described by Cate in relation to her father's departure without saying goodbye to her. In the last session reported, she also recognised messing up everything (possibly in order to destroy meaning). A movement towards integration is present in the first session reported from the third year of psychotherapy. 'She felt lonely and decided to meet her boyfriend': here, a clear connection appears between an emotion and an action. Cate expresses gratitude and concern for the analyst ('please do not get sick'), and directly or indirectly, she expresses her need for analysis and its usefulness.

Jasmine

This patient also starts off the first consultation by showing disconnection: a sense of urgency which is both shown in her behaviour and emotionally conveyed to the analyst, as she 'soon disappears without a trace'. This sense of urgency is also conveyed at the end of the consultation and disappears just as rapidly. Still in the first interview, Jasmine also states that she 'never knew' whether sharing private jokes with her brother when friends were present was pleasurable or embarrassing for herself or even more so to him. She also shows disconnection between professional fulfilment and a deep sense of futility that has no obvious reason. Her thoughts are communicated as external to herself. Her motives for entering analysis are also obscure, to the point that the analyst finds herself wondering, 'what does this articulate, thoughtful woman need an analysis for?'[3] Failure of integration, and efforts towards integration, appear in the clearest way in the appearance of all sorts of physical symptoms and ailments after six years of analysis: tinnitus, hypertension, tachycardia, then the development of breast cysts with the ensuing fear of cancer. On a psychic level, only a 'mute discontent' can be perceived.

The developmental history constructed in analysis is that of an unsatisfactory relationship with a mother who is described as offering no physical affection, and even worse, as being poorly capable of accepting and transforming suffering and negative feelings. Besides the patient's descriptions, this is felt strongly by the analyst in the countertransference, particularly when she feels (to her astonishment) 'strong dislike' for the image of a baby feeding at the mother's breast. The child seems to have sought a solution through a strong relationship with the father, which is probably linked to her high professional success; aspects of the unsatisfactory primary relationship with the mother, however, surface again in reported episodes of not being seen and not being appreciated by male figures such as a cousin in childhood and Mr K in adulthood: an appreciation that she had passionately longed for.

Lack of integration, however, is seen by the analyst (at least in some points) as due to defensive manoeuvres. Physical symptoms are viewed as a way to 'retreat to a narcissistic state of mind' where no object can injure or offend her. Later on, the physical symptoms are attributed with different defensive meanings: Jasmine filled her ears with loud noise 'in order to block out the voice of what she felt to be a dangerous seduction.' To turn off the 'loud noise' she was hearing in the transference, she turned to illnesses. Moreover, Jasmine's idea of having a second and a third medical opinion when confronted with objective data, such as the result of a biopsy, has the flavour of disavowal of reality, forging disconnection from a realistic fear for her health. Early traumatic experiences can be viewed as 'split-off' in an active manner, so that splitting appears not (only) as an effect of trauma.

Though I tend to favour a view of physical symptoms as mostly due to the incapacity to reach a different, more 'mentalised' form of expression, and as an effort to communicate in spite of this disconnection, I believe we cannot exclude that in some instances physical symptoms may be due to defensive operations. This can only be decided by the analyst involved in the specific case on the basis of the analysis of transference/countertransference dynamics. Grotstein's proposal, as outlined above, may be a useful way of bringing the two dimensions, defences and levels of integration, together.

JÖRG FROMMER

Freud's biological perspective

The onset of modern neuropathological research in the last quarter of the nineteenth century influenced Freud's thinking more than any other scientific approach (Frommer and Tress, 1993). Taking this into account, it is not surprising that already in his early book on aphasia Freud frames his own theory in relation to the argument of the English neurologist Hughlings Jackson. His stance was that neuropathology in general would uncover the fact that ontogenetically, as well as phylogenetically, older structures of the brain that are relevant for psychic processes are superimposed with younger structures, and that in the case of what Freud calls '*functioneller Rückbildung*' ('Dis-involution'; Freud 1891/1953, p. 89), the structure that is developed later and is more highly differentiated disappears, while the older and less differentiated structure remains. Later in Freud's life, after he observed that his case reports could be read like novels (Freud and Breuer, 1895d), he became convinced that damage to higher differentiated brain centres would cause *negative symptoms.* He argued that if the higher differentiated brain centres are not available to inhibit the less developed brain centres, this would stimulate *positive symptoms* as the expression of the disinhibited lower brain centres. Moreover, he extended the application of this principle to the field of psychic functioning through his concept of *regression*. Even today, the concept of regression is central to psychoanalytic theory in linking defence mechanisms to different levels of psychic functioning.

Why and how the neurobiological and the psychic levels of human beings are interconnected to each other was not of paramount interest for Freud. As a physician, he knew that it was absurd to talk about psychic life without taking into account the body and especially the brain. But as a well-informed reader of Kant and a student of Brentano, Freud also knew that psychic functioning follows its own rules, despite having many parallels with somatic processes. Even today, at least from my perspective, abstract ontological discussions about the mind-body relationship do not resolve the main clinical questions of psychosomatics.

My personal view on this subject combines a rigorous dualistic stance regarding methodology with ontological scepticism. In terms of *methodology,* and very generally speaking, qualitative understanding in humanities depends on hermeneutics, whereas causal explanation in science is based on counting and measuring according to quantitatively defined natural laws. This methodological hiatus inextricably implies that we have no secure access to ontological reality: the 'thing-in-itself', according to Kant, remains always outside of our knowledge of the world.

From semiotics to interpretations in social interaction

From a clinical point of view, one of the most interesting issues in this context is how patients communicate their regressive experiences to the analyst, and how the analyst is able to obtain access to these unconscious, irrational, and affect-driven experiences and needs. Obviously, the theory of *semantics* of ordinary language is too narrow for this endeavour because of the need to consider messages which may not be characterised as fully symbolic. In the mid- to late-twentieth century, *semiotics* began to have an impact on psychoanalytic thinking, with the works of Ferdinand Saussure in French-speaking Switzerland and France, Charles Peirce in Anglo-American thinking, and Karl Bühler in German-speaking countries. Bringing these accounts into a 'trans-theoretical' approach, I'd like to distinguish a theory of *symbolisation capacity* that works on a continuum between *pre-symbolic interaction* on the basis of physical exchange on the one hand, and *reflexive symbolic interaction* on the basis of verbal exchange on the other.

From the perspective of psychosomatic work, it is important to recognize that the primitive stages of this continuum involve the body, especially the instinct driven needs of hunger, desire, aggression, which are expressed in human behaviour in the form of physical interactions such as eating, snuggling, hitting, and in pre-verbal gestures and sounds that are closely combined with the excitation of the autonomous nervous system. In the primitive state, it is important to recognise that the *link* between the symbol ('*signifiant*' in de Saussure) and the thing which is represented by the symbol ('*signifié*' in de Saussure) is not established, so that primitive pre-symbols are restricted to the dëictic function of pointing to something whose meaning is dependent on the context in which it is used ('*Zeigefunktion*' for Bühler, 'index' for Peirce).

During the twentieth century, very generally speaking one might say that theories of human behaviour were characterised by a move from biology to semiotics and semantics, and from there to thinking about the human condition within social contexts, leading to Jürgen Habermas's thesis that psychoanalysis's understanding of itself as a natural science is a self-misunderstanding (Habermas, 1972). Today, behaviour that is directed by the highly developed cortical areas of the brain is seen as human action that uses symbolic functions in social contexts – it is the capacity to represent and psychically recollect the external world. Interpretation is a core activity at the symbolic levels of human action, and it inevitably involves ascription and presumption because our knowledge about the world and about other people is always restricted and incomplete. Taking this into account, we are faced with the fact that every communication starts with an assumption – or in psychoanalytic terminology with a *projection* – of what the other participant(s) mean(s). Successful communication can be distinguished from deficient communication, since successful communication is aware of the incomplete and tentative nature of its interpretations, whereas deficient communication is not. Thus, communication on the highest levels of symbolic interaction can be understood as ongoing processes of interactive interpretations of the world and other people, which work step by step to integrate different parts of the world and different perspectives on these parts of the world.

Symbol and symptom

Psychoanalysis relates to the aforementioned theories of symbolic development in two ways. On the one hand, psychoanalysis has had an impact on biological, linguistic, and sociological thinking throughout the twentieth century. On the other hand, the advancement of psychoanalysis through this period was influenced by theoretical developments in the humanities. Psychoanalysis is interested in linguistics because of the phenomenon that whenever communication processes on the higher levels of symbolic interaction fail, lower levels take over the leading role, including the activation of pathological innervation patterns driven by unconscious affects. Franz Alexander was one of the first who spelled out this interrelation, leading to his theoretical approach to psychosomatic disease which was ordered according to types of inadequate innervation patterns of the autonomic nervous system (Alexander, 1965). With his concepts of '*Desomatisierung*' and '*Resomatisierung*', Max Schur (1955) added a developmental perspective. He observed that under the pressure of unsolvable psychic conflicts, adults regress from functioning at higher levels of symbolisation to more primitive childlike modes that involve the body as an organ of expression of their nonverbalised needs, and this may finally result in psychosomatic disease.

One of the main contributions of psychoanalytic thinking to the theory of symbolisation is that primitive and more highly developed modes of mental processing do not exclude each other. Freud's differentiation between primary and secondary processes allows for the conceptualisation of both processes as working in parallel and defines psychic health in terms of the balance between them. Freud conceives of psychic illness as an imbalance of these two modes of psychic functioning. Considering that phylogenesis, ontogenesis, and psychopathology follow the same rules in order to develop a system of meaningful symbols, one could say that the psychic structures in primitive cultures, in children, in artists, and in the severely disturbed (e.g., psychotic patients), show a dominance of unsymbolised primary process activity. While the dominance of primary processes can be characterised by extensive loss of control over instincts and affects, the psychic structures of 'well educated' adults in 'highly civilised cultures' and in neurotic illnesses are characterised by an overdevelopment of the secondary processes, resulting in the suppression of needs and emotions. It should be noted that these mental positions are open to change: one person may find a well-functioning balance between satisfaction of needs and drive control under relaxed and well contained social circumstances but may regress to a state in which unintegrated, non-symbolised excitement breaks through in situations where there is a loss of a holding environment.

In this context, we could say that psychic and psychosomatic symptoms are caused by: (a) over-excitement and under-suppression of primary process forces, leading to anxiety and bodily symptoms, which express an over-stimulation of the sympathetic part of the autonomic nervous system; (b) an over-suppression of primary process forces and affects, resulting in depression and bodily symptoms of a sympathetic under-stimulation and a para-sympathetic-overstimulation; (c) the discordance of over-excitement combined with over-suppression of primary process forces, which results in bodily symptoms that indicate high excitement in 'normal' persons who on a conscious level see themselves as not being under pressure. Anxiety and depression take different shapes at different levels of integration. Anxiety that is close to the secondary process is characterised by moderate bodily excitement and restriction to certain situations and certain phobic themes, while in general believing that one's own existence is safe and under control. In contrast, primitive anxiety at the level of the primary process overflows all borders and is expressed by massive excitement along with the fear of loss of control and physical integrity. Correspondingly, depression shows a spectrum from mild feelings of being hurt and neglected by significant objects without somatic symptoms, to the complete loss of inner objects, libido cathexis of the ego, stagnation, anhedonia, and somatisation (Frommer, 1996; 2015).

Unconscious defence mechanisms also take different shapes at different levels of integration. Mature defence (e.g. repression, displacement) is characterised by intrapsychic functioning on higher levels of psychic integration, combined with emotions accessible for introspection, whereas immature mechanisms (e.g. projective identification) characterising lower levels of functioning, often involve somatic dysfunctions and interpersonal enactments, and are often solely accessible as countertransference.

Along these lines, in his early work Küchenhoff differentiated between three levels of psychosomatic disorders. He claimed that: (a) *psychosomatic disorders on the level of psychosis* refers to patients with symptoms of low ego-strength, impaired defence mechanisms, and a restricted capacity to symbolically express themselves; (b) *psychosomatic disorders on the borderline level* refers to patients who dispose with – or distort – representation of the external world and display archaic hysteric affect; (c) *psychosomatic disorders on an object relation level* refers to patients with symptoms which can be understood as some sort of primitive primary symbolic (Küchenhoff, 1992).

Jasmine and Cate

According to my interpretation in Chapter 2 of this book, due to regression in the analysis of Jasmine a sense of fragility emerged when she came into contact with her early traumata and her need for love and protection. This process was expressed by a significant change in the shape of her symptoms that had been mainly psychic up to this point: now she developed somatic symptoms as an expression of stress related over-excitation dysfunctions combined with hypochondriac anxiety. In terms of our attempt to shed light on the concept of integration from a linguistic and semiotic point of view, this change could be understood as regression to a lower level of integration, using more primitive defence mechanisms compared with the neurotic ones that predominated prior to this.

The case of Cate is completely different. Her wish for psychoanalysis is based on massive fear of death caused by cancer. Hypotheses regarding causal psychological impact on her illness are arguable. What we know securely is, however, that the threat caused by cancer destabilised her tremendously. Her psychic functioning appeared to be regressed to a borderline or even pre-psychotic level, implying subtle challenges for bearing countertransference and therapeutic techniques.

Commentary

JACQUES PRESS

The very title of this chapter conjures up an opposition between two apparently incompatible theoretical perspectives. The term *defence mechanism*, in its classical sense at least, refers to a psychic mechanism – be it conscious or unconscious – actively put in place by the individual. On the contrary, the terms *transformation* and *integration* both imply a process that entails development within a progressive continuity, a process likely to succeed or conversely fail. So they fit in more easily with a monistic psychosomatic theory. Both authors develop their arguments within this field of tension. They are clearly in opposition to each other: Jörg Frommer adopts a dualistic stance, which in my view is not only methodological but also informs his discussion of the clinical cases in which he refuses to take into account the role of possible psychological factors in the onset of Cate's cancer. Luigi Solano, on the contrary, supports a fundamentally monistic conception: for him each system should be viewed both in somatic and in mental terms.[4]

Jörg opens his reflection by referring to the concept of regression that is rooted in biology, before outlining a theory of symbolisation based on linguistics, and more specifically on semiotics. He finally refers to Küchenhoff's work of connecting various levels of somatisation with various levels of symbolisation. This attempt at classification is somewhat reminiscent of the work of Marty who defined a spectrum ranging from 'well mentalised' patients on the one hand to operative patients on the other (Marty, 1976; 1980). For his part, Luigi puts to work the aforementioned tension between 'defences' and 'integration'. His discussion raises a key question: deficiency or defence? Like him, I prefer to think in terms of a failure of transformation or failure of integration affecting the nascent ego. I am indeed extremely reluctant to use the term 'deficiency' because of its countertransferential implications: is there not, in each and everyone, areas of the psyche in which the processes of transformation might have failed to various degrees and which would thus consist in areas of somatic fragility?

I also share Luigi's idea that some forms of splitting do not primarily result in defence mechanisms but are the direct outcome of early traumas; this is in keeping with Grotstein's position which I would like to discuss at more length. It is indeed especially important to link in a dialectical fashion the failure of integration on the one hand, and radical defence mechanisms leading to drive-related extinction on the other. When the nascent ego is exposed to a sum of excitation that exceeds its capacity for metabolisation, two interconnected series of phenomena that potentialise each other seemingly occur. First, traumatic splitting (which can be multiple, as Luigi points out) leading to a dissociation between intellectuality and affectivity. Second, an attempt to extinguish drive-related excitation at the root insofar as it constitutes a threat that the psyche cannot face. In other words, the failure of transformation, and the radical forms of defence against undifferentiated affects, are two sides of the same coin. Luigi's discussion of the two clinical cases highlights this complex interaction very well: using his terminology, both Cate and Jasmine show various degrees of disconnection between symbolic and non-symbolic systems on one side (this is what I call the traumatic side of the coin), the other being the radical defences against affects because they are unmetabolised as a result of the early failure in the relationship to the primary object. I will add that this has important technical implications: the analyst must consistently evaluate whether a visible defence is in fact as it presents itself, or if it may veil a failure of transformation, and vice-versa. To an external observer, a failure of transformation may be easily mistaken for a classical splitting mechanism.

Another important question related to the same topic and explored by both authors pertains to the various levels of symbolisation. Whereas Luigi leans on Bucci's work, Jörg relies on the developments of semiotics. Even though they use different terminologies and distinct theoretical frameworks, they seem to agree here on the crux of the matter. The indexical function (Peirce) or the dëictic function (Bühler) of symbolisation mentioned by Jörg Frommer could be envisaged as closer to the somatic level, which Luigi qualifies as 'A' in his contribution on the theme of symbolisation (see Chapter 8). Both authors consider that this basic level of symbolisation is tied to primary process as described by Freud (Freud, 1900). This is a point that I actually disagree on. In my view, the psyche's basic material is seemingly less differentiated than primary process and closer to what Freud refers to as drive motion ('*Triebregung*') after 1920. Several theorisations of this basic level have been put forward: originary process (Aulagnier, 1975), primary symbolisation (Roussillon, 1999), parcellary unconscious (Marty, 1980), to mention only these. My argument here has important clinical implications. One can interpret material emerging from the primary process in terms of desire (and of the defences put in place against it); but one cannot directly interpret unsymbolised material, one can only help the patient give him a more symbolised form.

That said, to conclude I would like to point to two key elements which, despite their lack of formulation, operate as a silent backdrop and influence the approach of both authors as well as mine. The first one pertains to something that seems to be missing in both contributions. I am referring to the pivotal importance of the economic viewpoint. What are the active forces compelling integration or disintegration and which preside over or lead to the failure of the implementation of the various defence strategies which human beings have at their disposal? Based on my exchanges with both authors, I know that Luigi and Jörg are very critical of the concept of drive, which has an epistemological fuzziness and philosophical tone that they deplore. I personally remain attached to this concept. Indeed, pending the advent of a new paradigm that I myself wished for at the beginning of this discussion, I think we have not come up with anything better to theorise the psyche and soma in their unity and to understand the forces likely to lead to somatic illness.

My second silent operator becomes manifest thanks to the following question: what does it mean to be a psychosomatician? To me, it is linked to an ethical position. Being a psychosomatician does not consist in regarding some people as 'psychosomatic patients' on the one hand, and others as 'normal' individuals on the other. Neither is it a matter of distinguishing between 'psychosomatic illnesses' and other illnesses that would be entirely unrelated. Being a psychosomatician implies, in my view, a consideration of human beings in their psychosomatic entirety. It also consists in striving to understand the way in which each individual's personal construction – including a developmental perspective in terms of integration as well as the implementation of various levels of defence mechanisms – interacts with the individual's personal constitution and can possibly lead to somatic illness. This attitude leads me to reject Alexander's position. This author indeed undertakes a shift – or rather takes a leap – from a psychoanalytic perspective to a physiopathological approach in terms of sympathetic and parasympathetic activity (the activity of the autonomous nervous system). In so doing, he causes a highly damaging confusion between two planes of conceptual understanding that each have their own tools. Our current knowledge is fragmentary at best but taking shortcuts will fail to solve the problems. What remains to be achieved, conversely, is a construction of the intermediate stages between these various planes – a worthwhile goal for future psychosomatic research.

Notes

1 I explicitly avoid reference to dissociation or integration between psyche and soma (which appeared inevitable in 1966), since this implies a dualistic stance: my position on the mind/body problem was stated at the beginning of Chapter 8. The notion of dissociation or integration between different entities can be maintained by considering a differentiation among different systems or levels, as outlined in Chapter 8 (primary/secondary processes in Freud, beta elements, alpha function, apparatus for thinking thoughts in Bion), provided that each system is viewed both in somatic and mental terms.
2 In the alexithymia theory (e.g. Nemiah, Freyberger and Sifneos, 1976; Taylor and Bagby, 2013), and in other contemporary authors (e.g. Damasio, 2003), a distinction is made between emotions – the neurophysiological and motor expressive component of affects – and feelings: the subjective, cognitive-experiential component.
3 Irene Ruggiero reported a similar situation with a 17-year-old girl who initially brought to the analysis as her problem only an incapacity to decide which music and which clothes she loved most (Ruggiero, 2011). The analyst was faced with a strong countertransference, which led her to think, 'What am I doing here wasting time with this girl who has nothing?' She eventually recognised that (similar to Jasmine's analyst), she had identified with a patient's internal object (mother) who refused to recognise her daughter's anxieties. Recognition of needs and of anxieties seem to be two close aspects of the same dimension.
4 For a detailed discussion of psychosomatic monism *vs* dualism, see Chapter 8 and Solano, 2010; Press, 2016.

References

Alexander, F. (1965) *Psychosomatic Medicine: Its Principles and Applications.* New York: Norton & Co.

Aulagnier, P. (1975) *La violence de l'interprétation: du pictogramme à l'énoncé.* Paris: Presses Universitaires de France.

Bion, W.R. (1962) *Learning from Experience*. London: Heinemann.

Bucci, W. (1997) *Psychoanalysis and Cognitive Science: A Multiple Code Theory.* New York: Guilford Press.

Damasio A. (2003) *Looking for Spinoza: Joy, Sorrow and the Feeling Brain.* London: Heinemann.

Freud, S. (1900) *The Interpretation of Dreams. S.E., Vol. 2.* London: The Hogarth Press.

Freud, S. (1953) *On Aphasia. A Critical Study*. Madison: International Universities Press, 1891b.

Freud, S. and Breuer, J. (1895d) *Studies on Hysteria. S.E., Vols 4–5.* London: The Hogarth Press, pp. 7–305.

Frommer, J. (1996) 'Grundlinien einer Systematik der Neurosen und Persönlichkeitsstörungen', *Psychotherapeut*, 41, pp. 305–12.

Frommer, J. (2015) 'Phänomenologische Psychopathologie, Psychoanalyse und empirische Evidenz – ein Syntheseversuch mit autoethnographischen Bezügen', in G. Dammann (ed.), *Phänomenologische und psychotherapeutische Psychiatrie.* Stuttgart: Kohlhammer, pp. 36–50.
Frommer, J. and Tress, W. (1993) 'Einige erkenntnistheoretische Implikationen der Psychologie der Objektbeziehungen', in W. Tress and S. Nagel (eds), *Psychoanalyse und Philosophie: eine Begegnung.* Heidelberg: Asanger, pp. 183–99.
Grotstein, J.S. (1997) 'Alexithymia: the exception that proves the rule of the unusual significance of affects', in G.J. Taylor, R.M. Bagby and J.D.A. Parker (eds), *Disorders of Affect Regulation.* Cambridge: Cambridge University Press, pp. 11–18.
Grotstein, J.S. (2008) *A Beam of Intense Darkness: Wilfred Bion's Legacy to Psychoanalysis.* London: Karnac.
Habermas, J. (1972) *Knowledge and Human Interest.* London: Heinemann.
Küchenhoff, J. (1992) 'Zur kommunikativen Funktion psychogener Körperstörungen', *Zeitschrift für psychosomatische Medizin und Psychoanalyse*, 38, pp. 240–50.
Marty, P. (1976) *Les mouvements individuels de vie et de mort.* Paris: Payot.
Marty, P. (1980) *L'ordre psychosomatique.* Paris: Payot.
Marty, P., de M'Uzan, M. and David, C. (1963) *L'investigation psychosomatique.* Paris: Presses Universitaires de France.
McDougall, J. (1989) *Theaters of the Body: A Psychoanalytic Approach to Psychosomatic Illness.* New York: Norton & Co.
Nemiah, J.C., Freyberger, H. and Sifneos, P.E. (1976) 'Alexithymia: a view of the psychosomatic process', in O.W. Hill (ed.), *Modern Trends in Psychosomatic Medicine, Vol. 3.* London: Butterworths, pp. 430–39.
Roussillon, R. (1999) *Agonie, clivage et symbolisation.* Paris: Presses Universitaires de France.
Ruggiero, I. (2011) 'Comunicazione inconscia e lavoro di controtransfert: Riflessioni su una consultazione con un'adolescente' ['Unconscious communication and countertransference: Reflections on a consultation with an adolescent'], *Rivista di Psicoanalisi*, 57, pp. 71–84.
Schur, M. (1955) 'Comments on the metapsychology of somatization', *The Psychoanalytic Study of the Child*, 10, pp. 119–64.
Smadja, C. (2001) *La vie opératoire. Etudes psychoanalytiques.* Paris: Presses Universitaires de France.
Taylor, G. J. and Bagby, R.M. (2013) 'Psychoanalysis and empirical research: The example of alexithymia', *Journal of the American Psychoanalytic Association*, 61, pp. 99–133.
Taylor, G.J., Bagby, R.M. and Parker, J.M.A. (1997) *Disorders of Affect Regulation.* Cambridge: Cambridge University Press.
Winnicott, D.W. (1966). 'Psycho-somatic illness in its positive and negative aspects', *Int. J. Psychoanal.*, 47, pp. 510–16.

Conclusion

Jacques Press

Having reached the end of the collective adventure that was the writing of this book, let us take a minute to look back on it. It is commonly said that the path is made by walking, and these words are proven right once again: we certainly had expectations, but the path was unknown and, in some respects, only emerged *après-coup*. Two questions come to mind: what are the new elements that have arisen by our discussions on psychosomatics? And what are the cores of divergence over which we stumbled, despite the willingness to exchange that really was the driving force of our group?

I will start with the second question and address it with a point which, however anecdotal it might seem, remains highly revealing, all the more so since it concerns a central issue in psychosomatic theory. The sharpest discussions that took place among us were the ones in which the supporters and detractors of drive theory opposed to each other. The former not only stressed the centrality of the drive as a concept in the Freudian corpus, but also insisted on its necessity when theorising the somatic anchoring of the psyche, as well as the processes leading to somatic illness. Those who opposed the central role of the drive in psychosomatics foregrounded its vague and speculative character, its origin in outdated physiology and biology, as well as the multiplicity of diverging and often incompatible viewpoints among its advocates. The passionate nature of our discussions on this topic highlights a well-known fact, i.e. the considerable amount of narcissistic cathexis of our theoretical systems. This investment is probably all the more substantial since our theories serve as conceptual frameworks for our practice, whereas our discipline is not a *hard* science and thus cannot rely on a classical system of scientific verification. But this state of affairs further reveals the following: while it is true that we cannot dispense with theoretical frameworks, it is also true that we sometimes need to suspend these frameworks in order to exchange with authors of various orientations and advance knowledge.

This line of thought is undoubtedly reminiscent of a book by the great essayist Siegfried Kracauer, *History: The Last Things Before the Last* (Kracauer, 1969). Kracauer claims that philosophy is concerned with what he calls ‘the last things’: that is, with generalising, universalising theories of history. But ‘history’ seeks to explore what he describes as ‘the last things before the last’ – the specific, often overlooked elements of life, the world as discontinuous and ruptured. More specifically, Kracauer points out that *general theories* are commonly held to integrate the knowledge of *specific theories* – the kind of thinking that attends to the singular rather than the general. But, as Kracauer points out, *specific theories* see other things, not less things, and so they work in the cracks of the more general theories. Let us stress that this point of view pertains to an epistemological position, and not to any form of soft relativism.

Kracauer's lesson also fully applies to psychoanalysis and to our enterprise. It seems to me, in any case, that such was the path of the particular that gradually emerged as we made progress with our work. It led us to avoid debating the 'last things' directly in this book – whether they are the drives or the opposition between monism and dualism in psychosomatics – and instead we tried to remain, chapter after chapter, as close as possible to our practice and the questions it confronts us with. The fact remains that the 'last things' are bound to return at key moments as well as in the chapter devoted to drives and affects, which presents three different perspectives on this topic. But here again, the work is presented in such a way that the theoretical divergences at play do not take the form of outright opposition. What I want to stress is that a field of tension arose in (or along) this process, which in hindsight delineated our path: on the one hand, we strove to remain close to our practice and anchor our theoretical reflections in it, while going as far as we could to consider positions that differed from our own; on the other hand, we did not lose sight of our foundations, the foundations that we need in order to function as psychoanalysts and human beings: we cannot live without a frame of reference, it is in our nature.

Having said all this, we can now return to my initial question: what did we gain from our approach? One aspect emerges – and this applies both to working with each other in this book and to our work with psychosomatic patients – the experience of encountering another being who is at once similar and different, and acknowledging the limits of the encounter, can leads to new and potentially mutative avenues of thought. It forces us, admittedly, to clarify our way of thinking in order to be understood by the other. And the feedback given by the other sheds light on our own way of thinking. The outcome of this process is that we return to our own theories enriched with questions: we do not so much arrive at ready-made answers as at more complexity. This discussion may seem unconnected with psychosomatics. However, when one thinks about the difficulties often encountered in establishing a therapeutic relationship with somatic patients, it is highly significant: the issues raised in the *theoretical* encounters between us as authors actually resonates with the problems met in the *clinical* work with our patients and shapes the dynamics of our exchanges.

In this complex process, the ternary structure that we set up thanks to the discussant played a key role that we had not fully anticipated. This is the second important lesson we learned from our journey: that the dialogue between diverging viewpoints requires the introduction of a third in order to be productive; such is the role played by the discussant. This introduction of thirdness may seem quite obvious, yet it has been implemented very little in our field. We can see that the third takes on various forms throughout the book. The differences between authors are sometimes manifest, and the role of the discussant consists in foregrounding the basis of these differences, and at times highlighting the points of convergence veiled by the clashing theorisations. In other cases, the differences are much less evident. Two scenarios therefore appear as regards the discussant's role. In the first one, featuring more or less direct opposition, the discussant's role mainly consists in dialectising the different positions. In the second scenario, the discussant provides new and complementary elements. Let us point out that these two approaches had not been anticipated in any way, (nor is one more valuable than the other), rather they arose through the dynamics of our group and the writing process. One last comment on the subject. When the frame implemented by this thirdness functions optimally, something specific takes place – something whose import was visible to us during our discussions and which readers will find illustrated in numerous instances throughout the book. What unfurls then is a space of play which takes on a quality that we could characterise as transitional in the Winnicottian sense: these privileged moments have the merit of drawing our attention to an aspect that is too often overlooked: that the transitional space can only fully unfold provided that it is in a frame offering a *good enough* form of thirdness. Such moments are all the more important in our field, as our clinical experience often confronts us with situations in which transitionality is sorely lacking.

The third lesson to be drawn from our venture consists in the importance of the play of transference and countertransference in psychosomatics, where clinical situations are often stamped with negativity. The transference and countertransference are not only explored in the chapter dedicated to the subject, but they form a leading thread throughout the book; this path was not entirely unknown to us, and its outline emerged very quickly during our discussions. What is interesting is the specific forms that it took: the importance of the work on the analyst's pre-countertransference; the attention paid to transference and countertransference dynamics in somatic regression; attention to the bodily manifestations of the analyst; the emphasis placed in the psychosomatic investigation not only on the patient but on the initial dynamics of the analytic couple and not only on the patient; the emphasis on the dynamics between the analyst and patient and not just on the patient. All these factors lead us to question psychoanalytic theories of psychosomatics based on the idea that somatic patients are characterised as having *something missing*, which leaves them helpless before an analyst who is endowed with a much better psychic organisation, and that such patients are inaccessible to psychoanalytic treatment, short of major amendments to the setting. Our reflections outline a path for future work and research, which would consider the effects on the psychosomatic balance of these modalities of the transference and countertransference in which the two partners of the analytic relationship are fully involved.

A fourth lesson we gained pertains to our understanding of the somatisation process, and relatedly, to the work of symbolisation – from the somatic pole to the psychic pole. Our exchanges foreground this clearly, showing how somatic manifestations can be envisioned from two apparently conflicting viewpoints: as a failure of psychic work, or as *something* arising from the body that requires formalisation and transformation. The book also gave rise to the idea that thinking in terms of defence mechanisms is not enough in the psychosomatic field. This raises the following question: how can we maintain a binocular view? In other words, how can we move towards integration and transformation, while simultaneously retaining the active defences put up by the individual? Readers will have noticed that the authors' attempts at answering this question are diverse, leading to the re-emergence, once again, of 'the last things', with the opposition arising between those who support the concept of the drive and those who refute it. This marks the emergence of another potential research path, which would consist in forming dialectical connections between these divergent viewpoints. Finally, in chapter after chapter of this book, it seems to me that there emerged that the notion of a psychosomatic crossroad where various elements converge: the specifically psychosomatic effects of trauma on a psychesoma lacking the maturity to implement defence mechanisms (projective ones, for example); forms of depression that are not limited to essential depression, but are related to the Winnicottian breakdown or to particular forms of melancholia; disorders in the formation of psychic agencies, in particular the ideal ego and superego. A collaborative research project, where analysts working with somatising adults join up with child analysts focusing on the early relations between mother and baby, could open up very interesting work.

Generally speaking, this book as a whole can be read as a plea to consider human beings in their unfathomable psychosomatic unity, and to dispute the division between a psyche on the one hand and a body on the other. This is indeed the direction in which psychosomatic thought has been heading from the outset, but psychoanalysts still have a long way to go along this path. The road is equally long on the medical side. Modern medicine is highly effective and extremely technical, but it tends to reduce the human body to its mechanical dimension and to handle it in a way that can be qualified as operative. Dare we then dream of a future where the two movements of psychoanalysis and medicine converge to foster a new kind of psychosomatics shaped by generations to come?

Reference

Kracauer, S. (1969) *History: The Last Things Before the Last.* New York: Oxford University Press.

Index

Abandonment anxieties 63, 67, 103
acting-in in the soma/body 5, 13, 22, 68, 86, 90, 128
acting-out 5, 61–62, 64, 68
affect 7, 53–54, 104, 108, 109, 140, 145–46; affectless 35, 53; affect regulation 53–54, 58; and countertransference 104, 106; cut off from 40, 42, 43, 69, 107, 147; defences against 147; *désaffectation* 140; disqualification of affects 65, 106; and drive 100, 104–11; excess affectivity 88–89; primitive affects 140; 'quota of affect' 104, 110; and representation 86, 104–15
Aisenstein, M. 2–3, 13, 41, 53, 84–85, 88, 93, 99, 117, 133
alexithymia 40, 42, 46, 124, 139, 149, 150
alpha function 57, 102–3, 109
anality 5, 63
anxiety 16–19, 25, 49, 53–58, 65–66, 75, 127, 129, 145–46: automatic anxiety 65, 106, 108; bodily anxiety 126–27; diffuse anxiety 36, 38, 52, 86; massive anxiety 36, 38, 145; primitive 145; realistic anxiety 55–56
après-coup 63, 88, 151
association 21, 118
associative thinking 47, 78, 133
Aulagnier, P. 148

Bergeret, Jean 5, 63, 66–67, 69
beta-elements 6, 100, 101–4, 109, 116, 123, 125, 140
Bion, W. 2, 6, 37, 39, 57, 74, 78–79, 81, 129; *Cogitations* 101; *Elements of Psychoanalysis* 101; emotional storm 83–85, 93, 100; *Learning From Experience* 101; preconception 105; *A Theory of Thinking* 101–3; *see also* beta-elements
body: projection into 2, 5, 42; language of the body 6, 21, 64, 75, 87, 121, 126, 129, 132, 136; maternal body 120; *see also* acting-in
borderline 1, 5–6, 60–69, 74, 76, 80–81, 146
Britton, R. 39, 116, 117
Bronstein, C. 2, 41, 103
Bucci, W. 6, 124–25, 135, 139, 147

catastrophising 44
containment: analyst's 44–45, 88, 121, 137; container/contained 103; ego as container 114–16; failure of maternal 39; poor/lack of 62, 93, 124, 135, 140–41; in somatic symptom 117, 119; in the split 57, 58, 114; symbolic 53; uncontained excitation 68, 87, 113
countertransference 3–6, 13, 16, 19, 21, 23, 32, 35, 37, 39, 42, 44–45, 49, 52, 54, 58, 66, 68, 74–75, 78, 80–81, 83–85, 87–90, 92–95, 104, 106, 108, 110, 117, 119, 129, 131–32, 136, 138, 141–42, 146, 153
Cremerius, J. 73, 74, 77, 80

David, C. 2, 73, 76, 124, 139
De M'Uzan, M. 73, 76, 88, 124, 139
De Toffoli, C. 94, 123, 126
death drive 6, 40, 51, 92–93, 104–6, 109
death: fear of 56
defence mechanism 113, 115, 143, 145–46; manic defence 37, 39, 79; primitive 146
deferred action *see après-coup*

depression 4–5, 29, 35–46, 50–51, 57, 61–62, 66, 107, 117, 145, 154; melancholic depression 40–41, 43, 45; *see also* essential depression
destruction: of mental functions 40; of the object 53, 113
destructiveness 29, 39, 45, 56, 58, 61, 86, 105–6
diagnostic approach 6, 37, 44, 74, 78
disobjectalising function 46, 51
disorganisation 36, 38, 76; progressive disorganisation 40, 48, 51; *see also* psychosomatic disorganisation
dissociation 125, 137, 138, 139, 140, 147, 149
dreams 28, 30–31, 37, 43, 69, 104, 117–18, 126, 135
drive 39, 99–101, 104–6, 109; and affect 100, 104–11; drive theory and object relations theory 114; drive overflow/ excess 44–45; Freud's late drive theory 2; ego cut off from 5

ego ideal 6, 112–16, 120
emotional storm 83–85, 93, 100
emptiness, feeling of 27–28, 73, 133
Eros 86, 105
essential depression 5, 35–37, 38, 39–41, 43, 44, 50–51, 62, 154
evacuation 37, 44, 107, 114
excess/ too much excitation: 5, 45, 47, 52–53, 62, 68, 88, 102
external reality 5, 51, 57, 79, 130, 136

failure *see* containment and object
Fain, M. 2, 121, 131
fantasy 15, 23–25, 28–29, 41, 50, 55–56, 126, 140; of fusion with object 112; hallucinatory satisfaction 64, 109, 131; primal scene 65, 108; primitive fantasy projected into body 2, 5, 42
fear of breakdown (Winnicott) 2, 5, 35, 36–37, 39, 44–46, 52, 57, 79, 154
Ferenczi, S. 2, 47–48, 61
Ferro, A. 113, 124
Fliess, R. 63, 66
flight 5, 35–37; into sanity 37, 44
Freud, S. 2, 47–48, 52, 54–55, 123; 'compulsion to repeat' 47; beyond the pleasure principle 178; biological perspective 142–43; countertransference 84; drive 100–6, 109–11; ego ideal 13, 120; fear of death 56; fetishism 77; guilt 121; ideal ego 112, 120; 'Instincts and their Vicissitudes' 100; narcissistic cathexes 51; 'Mourning and Melancholia' 41; 'mysterious leap' 86, 99–101; *Papers on Metapsychology* 100; primary processes 148, 145; *Project for a Scientific Psychology* 102; 'quota of affect' 104; representation 130; secondary processes 124, 145; superego 116–17, 120; *Three Essays on the Theory of Sexuality* 99–100, 102; *Totem and Taboo* 129, 136; transference 83

Green. A. 58, 100–1, 105; acting out 130, 136; borderline state 60, 65–67; death drive as disobjectalising 51; drive theory and object relations 46; 'Primary Anality' 63; transference 86
Grotstein, J. 140, 142, 147
Gubb, K. 88–89

Habermas, J. 144
hallucination: hallucinatory satisfaction 64, 109, 131
hate 108, 115
Heimann, P. 74, 84–85, 87, 93
helplessness 21, 49, 131
holding 54, 91–93, 124, 128, 145
hyperactivity 37, 39, 44, 79
hypochondria 16, 17, 22, 48, 55, 75, 108, 118, 134, 136

ideal ego 58, 61, 68, 86, 93, 112–16, 120, 154
idealisation 16, 55, 66, 85–86, 93, 115, 136
identification 13, 16, 40, 54, 85, 91, 106, 108, 113, 116, 134, 145
internal objects 52, 57, 103, 113, 136
introjection 54, 66, 115
investigation *see* psychosomatic investigation

Kant 143
Kernberg, O. 5, 66–67
Klein, M. 2, 40, 43, 116
Kracauer, S. 151–52
Küchenhoff, J. 3, 146–47

Lacan, J. 2
language *see* symbolisation and language of the body
loss 13, 39, 41, 44, 49, 52, 57, 65, 145; early traumatic 50–51, 58, 114; of cathexis of body 56; significant object loss 29, 50–51, 66, 68; *see also* object

Marty, P. 2, 7, 40, 44, 48, 50–51; 69, 76, 78–81, 85, 88, 99, 124, 139, 150; operative life 35–37; operational thinking 66, 73–74, 147–48; *L'ordre psychosomatique* 78
maternal function 50, 76, 78; *see also* loss
McDougall, J. 2, 39–40, 50; *désaffectation* 140
memory: *see* screen memory
mentalisation (Pierre Marty's) 7, 51, 53, 56, 62, 76, 89, 110, 113–14, 122, 124, 131
mother-infant relationship 39, 62–63, 87, 89, 90, 92, 102, 126, 131, 132
mourning 41, 43, 45, 50, 57, 116

narcissism 38, 61, 66, 68, 77, 79, 89, 92, 103, 107, 121: borderline pathology 63; fragility 16, 22, 75, 81; narcissistic defences 113; narcissistic deficiency 80–81; narcissistic equilibrium 54; narcissistic investment 26, 51, 127; narcissistic trauma 50–51, 58, 81; narcissistic wound/injury 40, 74, 76–77, 79; omnipotence 86, 93, 112, 114, 120; primary narcissism 50–51, 58, 68, 81, 86–87, 112; retreat 131, 142
negative countertransference 106
negative transference 40, 58, 115
not enough of symbolisation 52–53, 56
Neyraut, M. 80, 83

object: failure of 21, 38–39, 44–45, 53, 57, 75, 92, 147; significant loss of 29, 50–51, 66, 68
objectification 66
oedipal: complex 11, 81, 108, 113; functioning 37; organisation 53, 58, 108, 115; development 63, 113; superego 68, 120
Ogden, T.H. 61, 125
omnipotence 28, 86, 93; narcissistic 112–15, 120
operational thinking 53–54, 66, 73, 77, 80, 88, 108, 147; *see also* operative life
operative life 7, 35, 36, 38, 44, 154; *see also* operational thinking
oral development 63–64, 120

paranoid-schizoid position 40, 125, 135
Paris School of Psychosomatics 2, 5–6, 35, 40, 69, 73, 80, 86, 88–89, 99–100, 103, 131
Pensée opératoire see operational thinking and operative life
perception 5, 47, 51–53, 57, 61, 89
persecution 41–43, 46, 58, 62, 120, 125; by ideal ego 112, 113; by object 39, 45, 46, 124, 136; by over-excitation 46; by superego 56, 117–19; by trauma 113
pleasure principle 86
pre-symbolic 56, 144–45
primary maternal preoccupation 78
primitive body: *see* body
projection into body: *see* body
projective identification 106
psychosomatic: disorganisation 50–51, 56, 58, 73, 114; equilibrium 2–3, 5, 42, 49–51, 54, 57, 130; investigation 2, 5–6, 36, 37–38, 67, 74, 76–80, 153; structure 53, 73–74, 77; symptom 2, 6, 39, 40–43, 48, 50–54, 57, 73, 75–76, 81, 85–86, 88–89, 104, 117–21, 134–37, 143–45

Racker, H. 16, 84–85, 87, 91, 93
reality: *see* external reality
regression 17, 46, 48, 51, 56, 58, 86, 113, 114, 128, 143, 146–47, 153
repetition: compulsion to repeat 47, 61, 104, 114
representation 21, 58; deficits/failures of 28, 51–52, 62, 65, 67–69, 86–88, 101, 107, 112–20, 126; disposing with 146; and drive 101, 102–4; reinforcement of 127, 129, 132; secondary processes 130
reverie 75, 89, 92, 102, 124, 128
Roussillon 6, 64, 69, 80, 82, 113, 122, 130, 132, 136–38, 148, 150

Scarfone 100
Scharff, J. 89, 90, 92
screen memory 15, 49, 133
Segal, H. 118, 135–36
separateness 42, 56
silent observer 4

Smadja, S. 2, 48, 50, 58, 86, 88, 99, 124–25, 139
somatic: *see* psychosomatic and regression
Spinoza 123
splitting 47, 51, 57, 65, 81, 108, 113–14, 121, 134, 140, 142, 147
split-off 21, 40, 45, 55, 57, 58, 61, 63–64, 75, 87, 89–90, 92–93, 108, 114–15, 129, 139–40, 142
superego 56, 68, 116–19, 120
survival (psychic) 2, 18, 44, 115
symbolic equation 118, 136
symbolisation 118, 121, 123–37; not enough of 5, 52–53, 56; organic symbolism 2; primary 6, 130–32, 136, 148
Szwec G. 89, 92

Taylor, G. 2, 89, 124, 139
third 4, 57–58, 62, 65, 67, 91, 114, 132, 152–53
transference 3–6, 37–45, 54, 69, 75, 78, 80–95, 106, 108, 115, 117, 118–21, 133–38, 153; 'transference of no transference' 66; in the Two cases 16–17, 20–21, 23, 24, 29; *see also* negative transference
transitional object 43, 53, 57
transitional space 153
trauma 47–60: as early loss 50–51, 58, 114; as fixation 47; as loss of maternal function 50; as moral shock 48; as persecutory 113; primary narcissistic trauma 50–51, 58, 81

unformulated experience 123–24

vie opératoire see operational thinking

Winnicott, D. 'Psycho-Somatic Illness in its Positive and Negative Aspects' 139

For Product Safety Concerns and Information please contact our EU representative GPSR@taylorandfrancis.com
Taylor & Francis Verlag GmbH, Kaufingerstraße 24, 80331 München, Germany

www.ingramcontent.com/pod-product-compliance
Ingram Content Group UK Ltd.
Pitfield, Milton Keynes, MK11 3LW, UK
UKHW020206200926
475702UK00004B/639

* 9 7 8 0 3 6 7 1 8 1 5 5 0 *